Sony and Writers' Guild Award-winning writer and comedian Mark Steel is best known for his critically acclaimed BBC Radio 4 show *Mark Steel's in Town*. Mark has presented the BAFTA-nominated Mark Steel Lectures for BBC Two, and is a regular on BBC One's *Have I Got News for You* and BBC Radio 4's *The News Quiz*. He has also written several acclaimed books, including *Reasons to be Cheerful* and *What's Going On?* He has also written an adaptation of his critically acclaimed stand-up show *Who Do I Think I Am?* for Audible, which was released in 2021.

One Man's Adventures in Cancerland

The Leopard In My House

Mark Steel

Cheers from Leith

EBURY PRESS

UK | USA | Canada | Ireland | Australia
India | New Zealand | South Africa

Ebury Press is part of the Penguin Random House group of companies
whose addresses can be found at global.penguinrandomhouse.com

Penguin Random House UK
One Embassy Gardens, 8 Viaduct Gardens, London SW11 7BW

penguin.co.uk

First published by Ebury Press in 2025
This edition published by Ebury Press in 2026
1

This book is a work of non-fiction based on the life, experiences and recollections of the author. Names of people, places, and the detail of events have been changed to protect the privacy rights of others.

Printed and bound in Great Britain by Clays Ltd, Elcograf S.p.A.

The authorised representative in the EEA is Penguin Random House Ireland, Morrison Chambers, 32 Nassau Street, Dublin D02 YH68

A CIP catalogue record for this book is available from the British Library

ISBN 9781529941036

Penguin Random House is committed to a sustainable future for our business, our readers and our planet. This book is made from Forest Stewardship Council® certified paper.

MIX
Paper | Supporting responsible forestry
FSC® C018179

*This book is dedicated to Elliot, Eloise and Rae,
who, it has turned out, will have to put up with me
for a little while more.*

Contents

One

Mirror in the Bathroom

Around the middle of June 2023, while I was shaving, I noticed that one side of my neck was much bigger than normal.

Is there supposed *to be a large, solid, visible lump on one side of my neck?* I thought.

And then, because I'm a bloke of a certain age, I answered myself *Yes, probably* and ignored it.

Because the first thought, when you notice a large abnormality on your body, is to assume the mind has made a mistake. Any explanation seems more plausible than the body having developed a sinister condition. Maybe the reflection is distorted by an eclipse of the moon? Have I got my left gland mixed up with my thigh? Perhaps necks develop lumps like this naturally, as protection against vampires.

When I googled 'Why is one side of my neck suddenly much larger than the other?' most of the answers suggested glands do this to fight off an infection, so there's nothing to worry about. 'Unless it hasn't gone down after two weeks.'

After two weeks I told myself it had, sort of, gone down, in that it was only a bit bigger. So I called the doctor's at exactly 8am to make an appointment, the way you have to, in the same way that millions of people try and buy tickets to see Taylor Swift at the exact moment they go on sale.

I arranged an appointment for the following week, then went to France for a wedding and almost forgot about it.

The following week I was in the doctor's office, talking in the blokey way that men often talk to a doctor, saying, 'I'm sure it's nothing; I'm sorry for coming.'

He felt my neck and throat and said, 'Hmm, it could just be some tissue, but I'll book you in for a scan at the hospital.' Then I went off to play football.

Nearly two weeks later I hadn't heard about this scan, so I rang the doctor, where someone told me to ring the hospital. So I rang the hospital and heard a long message telling me if I went to the hospital I would have to wear a mask because of Covid. It was slightly disconcerting that the hospital wasn't aware the Covid restrictions had ended two years earlier, but I ignored that and eventually was told to press something like 1 and then 3, then 8 and 5, so I drifted off as you do during these messages while it was probably telling me to press 4 to have a baby and saying, 'Remember, your tumour *is* important to us,' and then the phone went dead. So I called again and pressed all the numbers again and thought, *This lumpy gland had better turn out to be life-threatening after all this.*

Eventually I spoke to a gloriously jolly radiologist who asked me to 'come in on Sunday morning, darling, we'll find a slot for you, sweetheart'.

I was only going for reassurance. I didn't have anything wrong with me; I felt fine.

So after the Sweden v. USA women's football penalty shoot-out, I drove to the hospital. I was asked to lie on a blue plastic bench, where they covered my neck in sticky jelly and the radiologist placed a machine on my throat that looked like an electric shaver from the 1970s.

She looked at the screen while continuing with the conversation – 'Was there much traffic this morning? Shouldn't be too bad on a Sunday, it's not been too busy today' – then suddenly her expression became still, and stern, like the face you see on an actor at the end of a soap opera episode: the one that says 'someone's in a LOT of trouble'.

She rolled the shaver and looked at the screen again, closely, quizzically, as if she was in a science fiction film and was getting readings that showed I wasn't human, then rolled it back a half-turn, concentrating quietly.

'It's very enlarged,' said the radiologist, 'it's very uneven, and hard. I'm booking you for a fine-needle aspirational biopsy.'

Biopsy? I thought. *But that's how cancer starts. It always starts with a biopsy.*

I wanted to say, 'You don't understand. I haven't really got anything wrong with me, I'm only here for reassurance.'

Suddenly her stern face vanished, she smiled and said, 'I'm sure there's nothing to worry about,' the way a sergeant says, 'It's nothing to worry about,' in a disaster movie as he's telling everyone they must not on any account go outside.

*

The next morning the local doctor called me and sent me a text that started with 'URGENT REFERRAL'.

All those times I'd been frustrated that I couldn't get urgency from the doctor, and now they were yelling that I was URGENT. I wanted to be lackadaisically forgettable again.

There would be a phone appointment with a doctor on Thursday, I was told. I was asked if I'd suddenly lost weight, if I had night sweats, if I couldn't swallow properly, if I was out of breath, if there was blood in my mouth, if I smoked, how much I drank. These were all unsubtle cancer questions, as obvious as a detective leaning towards you in a cell and asking if you have any evidence that you were alone at home on the night of the murder.

*

The doctor who called from the hospital was Russian. He asked all the same questions. He said it was very good that I had no symptoms. I said, 'I know this isn't something you can definitely answer but I have to ask, do you think I have cancer?'

He said, 'Not good. Chances not good.'

I froze. 'Do you mean the chances that it's cancer are not good? Or that MY chances are not good?'

'Chances,' he said. 'Chances not good.'

One issue I've often complained about is the habit of tennis commentators on the radio, who say, 'Oh, and he's hit that shot into the net.' I sit in the car yelling at the radio, 'WHO? WHO has hit it into the fucking net?'

This situation was similar. 'WHOSE chances are not good? Mine or the cancer's?'

'Ah hah, yes, I mean unlikely you have cancer. But why you mention tennis?'

The biopsy would be within the next week, he said, and the hospital would contact me quickly with a date for this appointment.

I called my daughter and said sentences such as 'I've got to go for a biopsy on the lump but it's not like a biopsy where they think it's cancer or anything, it's more just to see whether the lump might be cancer and it's not a lump type of lump but more of just a lumpiness so it's probably fine.'

My son was in Edinburgh, performing his show at the festival. He was in a 60-seat theatre and most nights had sold all the tickets; he called me most days afloat with optimism and satisfaction.

I didn't want to tread on that by replying, 'That's marvellous that you're having the time of your life. My news is I might have cancer.'

I would tell him, I decided, when I met him during my visit to Edinburgh about a week later. I told my agent and various friends about the lump, each time feeling a slight sense of failure, because a comic depends on leaving any audience feeling at least a bit jollier than they started. And there seemed to be no way of telling this without causing anxiety and worry and very little joy. I couldn't make these gigs work at all.

Maybe a cancer scare is more suited to authors of thrillers.

I met my son in the Mosque Kitchen, the canteen-style cafe opposite one of the centres of the festival in Edinburgh. He excitedly told me about his latest review and I responded by telling him I was going for a biopsy.

He was adamant it was unlikely to be cancer, there were so many other more likely explanations for the lump. Most likely, he said, was that it had been caused by the damp under the bath that had come through to the ceiling.

Though we were in different stages of denial, we both convinced ourselves this was the most likely explanation for the formation of a large tumour in my neck, and I wondered if I should cancel the biopsy and call a plumber instead.

For the next three days I absorbed the chaos of the festival, the unexpected shows, the impromptu lunchtime beers; I met performers I hadn't seen for years on the cobbles and parks of the city, but when I wandered on my own I wallowed in nostalgic whimsical lingering outside so many flats, cafes, corners, bars and makeshift theatres where poignant personal dramas had taken place. There was the bar once called Buster Browns where I first performed at the festival: an appalling piece of nonsense inflicted on not many people in 1983. There was the corner by the Red Box cafe where I had a momentous kiss that led to three years of travelling back and forth to Paris.

There were the theatres where I'd first attracted my own audience and had felt unstoppable, and another where I'd been awful and sold few tickets and one night the emergency door flew open during my show and a homeless man walked in and sat on the stage. There were so many innocuous-looking locations – a park bench here or a Sainsbury's there – that had witnessed a friendship or a romance being ignited or incinerated.

There was the police station where I'd stood with Arthur Smith as he got all his audience to stand outside at midnight singing 'Free Nelson Mandela', until an officer emerged to say, 'I think you've been misinformed as Mr Mandela is not being detained at this station.'

And the bar where Shappi, who I would later fall madly in love with, approached my 19-year-old son at 3am, who was chatting to a young woman with clear romantic intent, to give him relentless advice on birth control until he shouted, 'Shappi, please stop talking about my sperm in front of my dad.'

Halfway across the glorious Meadows, the park that you seem to have to cross to get from anywhere to anywhere, it occurred to me that I probably did have cancer and this could be catastrophic and yet I was cheerfully strolling to the same makeshift bars that I'd had all these adventures in, and everything was normal except that I might be about to disintegrate.

*

I'd watched two of my closest friends get cancer. In Edinburgh, Linda Smith and I were in a little gang with Jeremy Hardy, who I often shared a flat with. Jeremy adored Linda as a person and as a comic, and he accepted what was happening to her before I did.

I first met Linda around 1987, when I did a gig with her in Sheffield where she lived with her lifelong partner, Warren. I stayed in their flat and Yorkshire TV was experimenting with the first all-night television in Britain. So we sat up, astounded by something being on at 3am; it seemed as marvellously unnatural as an experiment in which the sun set in the east.

Sitting up until that time with someone is probably the quickest way to get to know them. She told me about coming from Erith, a small town dominated by concrete walkways by the Thames in Kent, about five miles from my home town of Swanley. Famously, she said it wasn't twinned with anywhere but 'did have a suicide pact with Dagenham'. She also loved how the local paper once announced that the competition to name the new leisure centre in Erith was won by the entrant who suggested 'The Erith Leisure Centre'. She loved the cast of everyday life and found them hilarious. She told me about her days in an apple pie factory, in which raw apple pies would drift up a conveyor belt into an oven. Once cooked, a huge door would open and the pies would start on their way back down towards Linda and her colleagues, who would have to inspect each pie and remove any that were flawed. One man, she said, every single time the oven door opened and the pies came out, would say, 'Here come the little fuckers.' By the end of the night we knew we'd be mates for the rest of our lives.

There was a glow about Linda that evoked a style of rebellion combining modern outrage with a nineteenth-century love of beauty. She reacted against the soulless square concrete of her home town, like the Impressionist painters that saw their art as a retort to the functional grime of the Industrial Revolution. Anywhere in the country she would suggest a cafe that would turn out to require a two- or three-mile walk but she insisted we went there because she loved the tiles or the crockery. She was an obsessive gardener and equally obsessive about jazz. She bought me Dexter Gordon's *Our Man in Paris*, which introduced me to a whole new world in which I'd fill cupboards with my own jazz discoveries. She loved cricket and anything that existed for its own sake, rather than displaying the ugliness of concrete necessity.

Linda was always at her infectiously funniest in natural conversation and I'm not sure I was ever in her company for an evening without at some point howling in pain from laughing. In the same way she became loved by audiences of *The News Quiz* and *Have I Got News for You*, as her jokes revealed her delight in the beauty of life and its objects, and her heartfelt contempt for bullies. Her following came together to a point where she was selling out theatres across the country, until one day she told me during a cheery chat on the phone that she'd been diagnosed with ovarian cancer. It was all a bit annoying, she said, because the initial smear had taken place four months earlier but the hospital in Newham had lost the results.

Her schedule was to have chemotherapy and then an operation to remove what remained of her tumour, 'and if that doesn't work,' she said, 'it's a trip to Lourdes to pray'.

She said it in such a matter-of-fact way that I believed for a few moments that everything would be alright, because there were plenty of options, including going to Lourdes to pray.

One day she said she was enjoying her shows more than ever, so she'd come off stage in a state of great contentment, 'then a few moments later I'd remember I had cancer and that would spoil everything'.

Sometimes several weeks would pass with no news, then we'd go for a drink or spend an evening at her house watching *Curb Your Enthusiasm* or a programme about finding ghosts that she thought was hilarious. And I'd assume I'd misunderstood and she didn't have cancer at all, or she had one of those cancers that just goes away and you forget you ever had it.

Now I wonder what went on during the quiet weeks. I guess these were the dark times, when the treatment was tearing her apart and she didn't want to socialise. If there was nothing to talk about apart from cancer, she'd rather wait until there was.

One day we were laughing about her old neighbours in Sheffield, who had sent her and Warren a cutting in which they'd been declared 'Aston Villa Fans of the Week' in the match programme. As I giggled she said, 'Oh, it's not good news on the cancer front.' The treatment and the operation had failed to destroy the tumours, 'so I think it will be a trip to Lourdes'. She chuckled.

Then I carried on in a state of confusion that I didn't wish to disturb. Confusion allowed for hope, whereas clarity probably wouldn't. It had been over two years since this cancer had been discovered and there were no obvious visible signs she was ill.

She was still on the radio and television, but there were still periods of silence where I guessed the difficulties were hiding.

One afternoon I spoke to Warren and said I'd come round that evening. When I arrived, he called upstairs and around ten minutes later Linda walked down, one step at a time, one arm hanging limply.

She greeted me joyfully, and I had to gather myself to smile naturally and not wear an expression that said, 'Oh FUCK, you really HAVE got cancer.'

We spent some time trying to chat like everything was

normal. She told me how angry she was that she'd heard a neighbour shouting viciously at his young son. Then we talked about Tony Blair, and a performance she'd seen of *Toad of Toad Hall* in which the actors playing Toad and Mole had had a fist fight on the stage, and then I said I'd see her soon, drove round the corner and stopped, then sat in the car without moving for about 20 minutes.

The next time I saw her, she was in the Whittington Hospital, only just conscious. One week later Jeremy called to say I should go to her house that day. A few of us were there, Warren acting as host and Linda in a bed, immobile. As she lay unconscious in her last moments, one by one we chatted to her, though her contribution to the conversation was, to be honest, disappointing.

She died just after we'd all left, as the greatest skill of any comic is timing.

She was my first lesson in the closeness of death, in which your everyday life is altered by someone's disappearance. Along with Jeremy, we met up about once a week, she always brought presents for my kids, she called me in despair because she'd been at a Labour Party event that ended with a ridiculous attempt by Labour leader Neil Kinnock to sing 'We Are the Champions'. It's not the spectacular that keeps people we've lost in our minds, but these everyday minor events and a continuous background of fun and kindness.

So many times since she died, I've wondered what Linda would have said about whatever was happening in the world, but never more than during these days of ultrasound scans and doctors proclaiming 'chances not good'.

But this is one of the selfish things about a close friend dying of cancer: they're not around to give you their advice when you think you might get cancer yourself.

It was the first time the potential of the situation truly landed on me. All those things that happen when someone has cancer, I could well be about to go through each phase of them. Operations, chemotherapy, hair falling out, telling people how many years I've got, losing half my weight, doing something to raise money, being told you're brave', and debates about who gets to speak at the memorial. I felt the possibility of all that in my stomach.

I continued across the park to meet some comics at a venue called the Underbelly, and pushed the looming cloud of cancer out of my mind.

The next day I went into town early, watched a show, met an old mate and cancer barely crossed my mind. I obviously didn't have cancer, I'd decided, because I was enjoying myself and feeling calm.

In such ways the mind swings from one irrational train of extremities to another. I told a few people about the lump, and didn't mention it to others. Whether I did or didn't wasn't affected by how close I was to them, it was down to my mood at the time.

One night I saw someone who works at my agency and immediately told them everything, but the next night I saw Matt Forde, the brilliant political impressionist, in his show and when we met for a drink afterwards we chatted about comedy, the Labour Party, how to do impressions, football. But when the break in the conversation came where I was about to say, 'Here, Matt, I've got this lump,'

I decided as it was a gentle August Edinburgh night that wouldn't have been enhanced by the introduction of cancer, I wouldn't mention the subject now throbbing through each corner of my head.

This was, by a long way, the most serious medical situation of my life. It was ten days since the biopsy would definitely be within the next week, so I rang the hospital, listened to the Covid message, pressed all the numbers, was put through to someone who told me I was someone else, and was left on hold, like a cancer version of when you ring Sky to change your TV package or call the shop that didn't deliver a fridge on the day it said it would.

When I finally got through I said I hadn't been given a date for the biopsy and was told, 'Right, so you want to come in for a scan.'

'I've had the scan,' I said.

'No, you haven't, that's why you're ringing for a scan.'

'I definitely had a scan,' I told him, 'I remember it in some detail. Then the doctor called and said I'd be called quickly about a biopsy.'

We went round this circle twice more, then he said, 'Oh yes, you need a biopsy, but we call a biopsy a scan, that's why you were getting confused.'

So I asked if he could give me a date for the biopsy/scan and he said that was done by a different department and they were all away.

A few days later a woman called who oozed weary compassion. She was so sorry, but this system can be such a mess and they haven't enough staff and she really did apologise but it's like that everywhere in this hospital at the moment. She gave me a date for the biopsy but then I'd have to wait four weeks for the results.

On the day before the biopsy was due, I was called by someone who said, 'Instead of waiting four weeks, you can come in on Saturday to discuss the results.'

'That sounds much better,' I said, 'but will you have the results that quickly?'

'No,' she said, 'they won't be ready.'

'What's the point in coming in to discuss the results, if you haven't got the results?' I asked.

'Do you not want that appointment, then?'

'Well, I do, but only if you've got the results.'

'I told you, we won't have them,' she said, and she was right – she had already told me that.

'I don't think there's any point in me coming then,' I said.

'Oh, Mr Steel', she said in a jaunty jolly voice, 'I wish you'd make up your mind.'

At the biopsy I lay on another blue plastic bench, my head facing the wall and covered in paper towels. I was asked questions about which doctor I had seen and why it wasn't the other doctor and when I'd had an endoscopy and questions that sounded like 'Has your biopetremedarist given your trisinomadon levels?' and 'Which Calvinologist measured your polyglutomas?'

I heard the doctor say to the nurse, 'Hmm, it says fine needle but I'll need the BIG needle for this.'

I wondered how big this needle was. In my mind it was five feet long, the sort Wile E. Coyote would use for capturing the Road Runner.

A few moments later I could feel the big needle sinking into my lumpy neck to extract the cells it needed, and the doctor said, 'Hmm, suspicious.'

There was a loud popping sound as the extracted cells were clicked tight into a tube to be sent away, and it was finished.

By now I was becoming familiar with the heightened tension in any room with a doctor that has any relation to cancer diagnosis. You become alert to the slightest facial change they display. The tiniest wrinkle of a nose sends you into a spiral of despair: *What did that wrinkle mean? They've discovered I've got no stomach. Look at the way the nurse is holding the pen. It's a grip that is consumed with the melancholy air of catastrophic news. I'm done for.* 'Very hard tumour,' the doctor said as I got up. It was hard to tell myself his comment didn't suggest I had a very hard tumour.

Now I would have to wait four weeks for the results, which would be presented to me in an office.

Was this to drive the drama to the maximum, as if the system was designed by Simon Cowell? As they're about to tell you the results, does a bass drum start like at the end of the *Strictly Come Dancing* results show? As the doctor is about to tell you, do they stop and say, 'But now we're going for an ad break. We'll be right back to reveal the results.'

But the doctor told me I wouldn't have to wait four weeks, as someone would contact me 'in around seven days'.

It's a wonderfully casual process, when you consider the results they're referring to could tell you whether you'll live or die. It's all said with the air of a decision about whether you can join a pottery class.

So the days after the biopsy were more terrifying than the biopsy itself. Every call from an unrecognised number stared at me with menace.

I would answer a call from an unknown number in a jittery, breathless state and say, 'OK, hang on, I just need a minute to compose myself, I'll take a breath – right, go on.' Then I'd hear someone say, 'Hello, Mr Steel, I'm Dave calling from Octopus Energy about changing your energy supplier.'

Several people had told me that if the results were ominous, I would hear quickly. So when five days passed, I felt confident.

At the local doctor's surgery, the receptionist gave me the results of a blood test I'd taken, on which someone had written 'normal', so that must settle it. The receptionist said there would have been a comment that the results were 'suspicious' if the cells were suspicious, so I was obviously fine and this lump was probably a piece of cheese that had become stuck in my neck.

Two weeks drifted by, then at a meeting with the Russian 'chances not good' doctor, I was told my biopsy was still being checked. I was booked in for an MRI scan and a CAT scan and I became aware of what someone had warned me, that cancer, or even potential cancer, can be a full-time job.

Just after I'd come off stage from presenting some awards in a hotel in Paddington, I looked at my phone. I'd received an email that said, 'We apologise for the inconvenience but your biopsy result was lost in transit. So you need to arrange to come in again for another biopsy.'

I strolled to the Underground in a trance. How could this happen? Had the system for taking biopsies to the testing centre been outsourced to Deliveroo? Maybe they'd mixed my biopsy up with some chilli sauce for a Mexican takeaway, and some poor sod had spread it on his burrito. Did I trust them to take another one? What would they do with it this time? They might send off a jar of pickled onions by mistake, then I'd be told, 'You don't have cancer but your blood contains an alarming level of vinegar.' A few days later the local doctor called to say they'd had another look at my blood test and decided it wasn't normal, but 'very suspicious'. Then a completely new person called me and said I had to go in for a repeat biopsy the next day, 'to see what stage of cancer you have'.

'Hang on,' I said, 'no one has said it's definitely cancer, are you saying it's definitely cancer?'

'Yes,' she said. 'Of course, that's why you came in.'

I sat still on the settee, numb and bewildered, and angry at the flustered manner I'd been told I had cancer, considering the many consequences of having a fatal disease, one of which is it would be fatal.

You're often advised, if you feel anxious or deeply upset, to try and locate where in your body you feel the emotion. But at the moment it was everywhere. There was a thumping in my stomach and a lightness in my head, and my legs tingled and my neck felt huge – and maybe guilty, as it seemed to be the cause of all this.

My generation was brought up thinking cancer was as final as being beheaded. If someone had cancer, to ask 'Will they be alright?' was as daft as replying to someone who'd said 'Alf's had his head chopped off' by asking 'Will he be alright?'

And as well as feeling the dismay of being told I had cancer, I had the ungrounded sensation that I couldn't trust the people responsible for dealing with the cancer.

*

So many appointments followed, in which I'd wander through this mysterious system of tunnels and lifts and pink zones and blue zones - corridors in which trolleys swing from unexpected side-turnings carrying someone with an oxygen mask, where cleaners and pharmacists and surgeons and radiologists coalesce to create this extraordinary factory of living, and that join rooms where fellow patients, staring on their seats, are awaiting calls into other rooms that haven't been decorated since 1983 to be told what their X-rays, scans and blood tests mean. As hundreds of patients flow through in the same way as you, you're all passed from receptionist to nurse to doctor to consultant as each staff member works through an endless list of people to care for. And many of the staff are paid appallingly and treated with contempt and their minister was sacked and went on *I'm a Celebrity* so don't take out your frustrations on them. And you're just one patient, so you need to be stoical.

A friend who used to be a nurse advised me it was essential to be a 'polite pest'. If you don't understand what they're telling you, you must ask. Politely.

I prefer to not be any kind of pest, but it's reasonable

to ask politely how they could have lost the biopsy and forgotten to tell me I had fucking cancer.

I was then called in to see a consultant, so I went with my son. As we arrived the doctor looked at his screen and said, 'I'm afraid it's not good news, Mr Steel.' You don't realise how much you want to live until a doctor in a meeting about cancer says, 'I'm afraid it's not good news, Mr Steel.'

The biopsy had been found at a different hospital and the results had come back from an MRI scan and a CAT scan and I had to go to another hospital the next day to learn the details, which he couldn't tell me, though he could tell me the lump was definitely a secondary cancer, which meant I had cancer in at least two places.

'Is this deadly?' I asked.

'Touch wood,' he said. And then he touched some wood, which I suppose was being professional.

Maybe if the scan results showed the cancer had spread to my lungs, they'd offer a more extreme approach and get me to pick up a penny and pass a black cat.

My head ran into a series of extreme areas. I was with Linda and Jeremy in their final days and often wonder about the sheer randomness of how long we're allotted. If I conked out now, would that be unlucky? I would still be luckier by several years than either of them.

I wondered if my son and daughter could carry on living in my house if I died, or would that involve me filling in a pile of complicated forms and trying to remember forgotten passwords? I wondered if it would be fair if my son had my car and my daughter had my record collection. I pondered what the jokes would be. Would someone say there's a new radio show called *Mark Steel's in Ground*?

I hugged my son (which he later claimed was 'the first time we'd hugged since the day Margaret Thatcher died'). I remember telling him he and his sister and niece were the people I cared about most and the main reason I wanted to live.

My granddaughter was a few days from her second birthday, which was perfect for the grandchild of a comic as you can bring back all your old material. I could do characters I thought I'd never use again, such as the always-hungry shark who threatened to eat all the furniture. And, because she wasn't quite two, she seemed to ignore the numerous flaws in the logic of this theatre. She and all the people close to me, going out in circles like ripples on a pond to the outer layers, people I exchanged occasional texts with but who were still joyful figures in the intricate plot of my life, all zapped around the landscape of my chaotic thoughts, that swirled with disorder as if they were the flakes of a snow globe that had been tipped upside-down and shaken more vigorously than ever before.

A moment like this certainly affirms what matters most to you. Because I don't recall thinking at any point 'I hope I don't die because I was looking forward to the iPhone 17 with the extra pixels'.

My son and I got in the car and he told me I should try and have a normal day, the day I would have had if this meeting hadn't happened.

We went to my favourite local cafe, where my friend Vissie is the manager. Later she said she knew from our expression as we went in that I was in a bad way. She gave me a hug and I said, 'I'm in a bit of trouble,' a phrase that in retrospect had less impact than intended as it was the catchphrase of the lovable 1970s sitcom idiot Frank Spencer.

I tried to have a normal day. I went to the Oval as I'd planned weeks earlier, to watch the cricket with two friends. At the very moment I arrived, it started to rain and the players came off, which seemed fitting, so we went to the bar. I told them what had happened and after they'd sympathised we discussed who was the greatest all-rounder out of Ian Botham and Ben Stokes.

Then I went to my weekly French lesson in which I speak French with the adorable Fatima. Forlorn and gaunt, I was explaining how the hospital had lost my biopsy, '*ils ont perdu le biopsie*'. With resignation she tapped me on the arm. '*LA biopsie*,' she corrected me, '*la biopsie est feminine*.'

*

I remembered when Jeremy first told me about his lump. The procedure to remove it was booked and cancelled again because of a show that was also booked in somewhere so when he got a new date we went for a curry because he wouldn't be able to have another one for a while after the lump was taken out.

A few days later he told me a consultant wasn't sure what the lump was but knew it wasn't cancer and we relaxed, him more than me I should think. I assumed this episode would only live as a routine in his next show. But he called a few days later as I was walking to the Co-op, to say it *was* cancer, of the oesophagus.

At that moment the signal cut out and it took three or four minutes to call back, as if the phone was directing a soap opera and leaving me on a cliffhanger.

He said there were parts of the scan the doctors didn't understand, and there would be more tests and there was something on his bones that wasn't cancer but they needed to work that out.

We'd first met at the Edinburgh Festival in 1984, then performed together at so many shows and at events for campaigns. We spoke at each other's weddings and we babysat each other's kids. We wrote radio shows and TV shows together, went to meetings about ideas for shows that would never happen, and when my son was 11, we went for a meal at Jeremy's house where someone asked him to pass the salad and he said, 'Get it yourself, you lazy cunt,' which made my son laugh for the next three weeks.

Jeremy campaigned forensically to help secure the release of people who were wrongly imprisoned, but one of the few moments he seemed genuinely pleased with himself was when he was in an office with a flip chart and he turned a few pages over and drew a huge cock and balls on one page, giggling at the prospect of some poor sod giving a presentation in the future and turning over the pages so all his colleagues would see this work of art.

Michael Gove once wrote an article in *The Times* saying that the two of us were on the radio too often, and an unofficial rule was agreed that we weren't to appear together on *Newsquiz*, as if we were a pair of mischievous children that had to be stopped from sitting together at school for our own good.

We went on holiday together and sat around each other's houses so many thousands of times, sometimes to drink tea or beer or whisky, sometimes to discuss one of our divorces and now to keep him occupied during his chemotherapy.

I was numbed when he told me he had cancer, truly numbed in that every sensation in my body was flattened. I couldn't feel myself; my sense of taste and smell and touch became a dull, sticky vagueness. I now had that feeling again with my own diagnosis.

*

I returned from my French session. My son's girlfriend was staying, which now seemed a little awkward. We chatted about her job and her love of Shetland, where she was brought up, and I popped into the conversation that earlier that day I'd found out I had cancer in at least two places but at least the consultant had touched wood so not to worry, then tried to carry on talking about how dark it gets up there in winter.

I tried to reach a more balanced view of my situation. I was convinced by someone who had recovered from cancer that there was a long way from here to a diagnosis that was terminal.

Most cancers now are seen as curable. Even the ones that aren't curable are treatable and patients live for many years.

In any case, it wouldn't help to panic. Whatever the cancer, there will be a plan to deal with the cancer.

She got out her violin and asked if I fancied playing the piano to accompany her in a couple of Shetland folk songs. So I did. My son looked as appalled as he was bewildered.

Two

Love Will Tear Us Apart

On the day I first felt my lump, I had no doubt who I wanted to share this experience with, to sit together with through the shocks and laughs and fears, the biopsies and cannulas that may lie ahead. The problem was I hadn't seen her for six months.

*

I'd known Shappi for many years, though we can't work out precisely when we first met.

It seems probable it was at a meeting called in opposition to the war in Iraq, where I was speaking with Tony Benn. She remembers asking if I was going to the pub, that I said I might, but I didn't go and on top of that the war in Iraq took place anyway.

So she had her picture taken with Tony Benn and we didn't meet again for a couple of years.

After that we were on the same bill many times, often at benefits, which are one of the main ways comics keep in touch with each other. We've all performed to raise money for a cause we've never heard of in order to talk to other comics we haven't seen for two years. Then you feel slightly guilty when someone from the charity you've just supported beams and says, 'Thank you SO much for doing this, we will FOREVER be grateful that you care so deeply,' and you're thinking, *I only agreed to do this so I could chat to Stewart Lee.*

Whenever we were on one of those bills, she'd amaze me with her expansive enthusiasm for something, anything, everything, and the exact words didn't matter. It was the manner of the words, the exuberance, the mischief, whatever the subject, arms waved at complex angles: what she said mattered to her.

Whenever I met her, she'd already be in an animated dialogue with someone; it could be an influential TV producer but was as likely to be a woman who worked in the baker's who, while she was wrapping a tuna sandwich, Shappi had persuaded to come with her to Glastonbury.

She could enthuse about Jarvis Cocker, take a perfect cutting from a plant, describing it as she went, tell the washing machine to shut up for beeping, explain the reason she was at that moment ordering a set of table mats online and do a perfect impression of her Glaswegian friend haughtily sending her kids to bed, all in one sentence.

After my marriage ended, we went for a drink and later that week for another drink and for a coffee, and met at odd times of day, just to be friendly. Our meetings were always frivolous and eager and we'd smile during the silences, and we'd fill in the gaps in our knowledge of each other's pasts, agreeing it really was awful how he/she treated you like that, each of us thinking, somewhere between the back and front of our mind, *You wouldn't get treated like that by me.*

Sometimes as we'd walk through a park or pop into the Post Office it felt so natural it was as if we were married, and I had to stop myself from holding her hand and asking if we were alright for cat food.

Then we arranged to meet in a pub one evening and sat by a chunky oak table in a dimly lit alcove that felt exactly like where you'd want to be if a nuclear bomb went off, relaxing until you caught fire.

She looked at me, with those fucking great eyes, right into mine, locking on to them like the most accurate of rifles on an Apache helicopter.

And I looked back into those eyes, and bits of me dissolved and I struggled to find any more words. Partly, I suppose, I knew I'd remember these words, so this was how Neil Armstrong would have felt if he hadn't prepared anything as he left the spacecraft to step onto the moon, thinking, *Shit, what do I say?*

Eventually I squeaked, 'Oh, we're in a pickle.'

I've no idea how powerful it must seem for those people who suddenly feel Jesus come into their heart, but I reckon it must be fuck all compared to the tsunami of emotion at that moment.

She was born in Iran, where her father was an acclaimed satirist and poet, a critic of the shah, the dictator who ruled her home country. But when the shah was overthrown, the country began to fall under the grip of the Islamic Revolutionary Guards, and what do you know, this lot was even more dangerous than the last and the family had to flee, so they came to London.

On the other hand, I'd recently discovered my biological father was a multi-millionaire former world backgammon champion, whose family fled from Egypt. They were Jewish, and under the rule of Gamal Nasser, tens of thousands of Jews living in Cairo left, as life was made extremely troublesome for them, following the bombing of Egypt by the British and Israelis in 1956. My father's family were among them.

Now there were times when I'd think, *Bless them all – bless the shah and the ayatollah and the British Empire and the Egyptian antisemites, because without them all I wouldn't be here with her in the kitchen, buttering her toast.*

We tried to fuse our lives together and half-managed it for a few months, but my kids were young and her kids were younger and she wasn't ready and I was busy and she was chaotic and I was chaotic, so we fell apart and kept in touch and fell apart and met up again and even when we weren't 'together' we'd look into each other's eyes and anyone watching would assume we went to Homebase together every Sunday morning. She would pick flecks of cotton off my shirt and I'd smile directly at her the way you only do with a tiny handful of people in your life unless you're very creepy and we went backwards and forwards like that for several years, unable to make it work to be together, but even less able to make it work to not be together.

We'd tried again and helped with each other's work and made each other's kids laugh. I sent her Willie Nelson's 'Valentine' and she cried a bit and she found the old picture of her and Tony Benn and realised I was prominently right behind her shoulder all along. We talked about where we'd have a wedding and walked her dogs and went to festivals and discussed the next 30 years, until one day she said she felt overwhelmed and called it all off and I was a tiny bit upset and a little bit fuming.

No schism in a relationship is really sudden, it just seems like it to the poor sod who didn't realise it was on the point of snapping. The other one has been smiling and going to the bar and chatting about the funny clips they saw on Instagram as normal, except it's not as normal because they're battling to appear calm while bursting with anxiety and confusion and a desire to ask for a pause in the demands of coupledom as they're feeling overwhelmed.

Inevitably in this situation, the person taken by surprise tries to argue their case, but I doubt whether anyone in all of history has managed to argue their way back into a relationship with logic. You can complain 'but you said a few weeks ago ...' or 'you're contradicting yourself again', but no one has ever said, 'You know what, you're right. Now I've seen your list of reasons showing why we should still be together, I realise my mistake,' as if it's a discussion about which gas supplier to change to.

But what was, I suspect, unique was that I was told all this in the week that we were supposed to appear together as a couple on *Pointless Celebrities.*

So we held it together for the day – not just held it together but won the jackpot, working beautifully as a team, Shappi with a series of brilliant answers about names for jewellery and American holidays and I had to think of 'pointless' answers to the question 'name anyone who has played Roger Federer in a Grand Slam final'.*

After that we didn't see each other at all, up to and past

* I went for Marin Cilic, Mark Philippoussis and Juan Martín del Potro. The first two were pointless and Del Potro scored one.

the cancer diagnosis, though for several months we communicated via angry messages to each other, the sort you would only write to someone you're in love with. I can't pretend to know precisely how the mind works during these periods of furious estrangement between two people in love, but I suspect part of your thinking is that you will seek to resolve it all eventually, after a sufficient period of annoyance has passed. After all, there's plenty of time. What's the rush?

Now one of the many typhoons that swirled through my mind after the biopsy result was that I might never see her again.

Two days before the ultrasound scan, she sent me a message that I ignored for a few hours. Then I replied but she ignored me for a few hours. Eventually she said she had something of mine that she wanted to bring round, that she'd told me in a previous message she'd put in the bin, so I agreed to meet her but she didn't respond and with hindsight we wanted to see each other so much that we both made certain we wouldn't see each other at all.

It all seems so infantile but the same emotions that prevent people from resolving these conflicts when you're 17 are still at work 45 years later. You fear investing any more emotion or hope into a situation that's already left you feeling battered, so you hesitate and wonder and rage and regret, and you keep in contact by effectively saying, *I desperately want you to know I still exist, not that I'm bothered if you know or not. And I desperately want to talk to you, to let you know I'm not bothered whether I talk to you or not.*

But this isn't ideal mental preparation for an ultrasound scan for a suspected tumour in two days' time.

Then I did the worst two things I could have done, which was to have a fling with someone else and get cancer.

It felt slightly comforting to go on dates, as it does when your heart is broken, and ideally someone from the council would have come round to put a stop to it, the way a boxing referee does with a fight that's a clear mismatch, but that wasn't possible with all the cuts that have been made to local authority budgets since austerity.

Then my date and I didn't see each other for a couple of months but met up again, probably because we were both a bit lonely. There are many books and websites that might advise what I should have said in a situation like that, but it's unlikely any of them would suggest the line I came out with, which was 'By the way, I've had an ultrasound scan and I think I've got cancer.'

So instead of a brief doomed affair with someone who would then be consoled by friends telling her 'he doesn't deserve you', I'd embroiled her in a cancer story. She must have felt like one of these characters in a children's book that goes into a sweet shop but it takes off and travels through space.

*

On the morning after the 'touch wood' day, I left the house again with my son, to travel to Tooting and discover my fate.

The most sinister aspect of this morning was how frighteningly unsinister it was. It was so normal. We drove through the early morning Streatham traffic with all the other motorists nudging forward and turning left or right as if it was a normal day and this felt so wrong.

We sat in a waiting room preparing for the results of my MRI and CAT scans. 'I just want one win,' I said. 'I feel like a football team that's nine games into the season and I've not had one win. Every meeting, every scan, it always gets a bit worse.'

My son and I chatted about football and comedy and the Labour Party, as all around us sat assorted patients with unknown ailments, and from this mundane setting I awaited this momentous news.

An hour late, my name was called. The doctor apologised, I said it was fine, fighting the urge to shout, 'Just tell us if I'm going to die.'

Like the Terminator assessing a biker in a bar, I made a series of calculations about the environment of this office. Did he look like someone about to say, 'You're completely done for, I'm afraid'?

Dr Oikonomou was Greek, maybe in his late thirties, with a smooth, compassionate manner. He seemed to want to smile, slightly. What did that indicate?

'The first thing,' said the doctor, 'is we have looked at the scans and there is no cancer in your lungs.'

'There's your first win of the season,' yelled my son.

I asked the doctor if he was a football fan. 'Of course,' he said. I explained why he'd said that, and he said he understood.

The scans showed the cancer was all restricted to the head and neck area, he said, and hadn't spread to a different region.

'Next I have for you a good draw,' he said. 'We think the primary cancer is a lump in your throat and that is very treatable.'

I suggested that was another win but he insisted it was a good draw.

Then there were some details about surgery and glands and chemotherapy and radiotherapy and PET scans and taking six months off performing but I didn't hear much of that as it was the moment I was assured I would probably live through this. He was sorry I would have to cancel some shows, but at that point I'd have been delighted if he'd said I would be alright although I would have to spend the rest of my life placing raisins into bars of Cadbury's Fruit and Nut. I looked to the heavens I don't believe in and sighed for two minutes.

'What team do you support?' asked my son as we left.

'Chelsea,' he said.

'Normally that annoys me,' said my son, 'but today that's absolutely fine.'

*

All emotions are on a spectrum, especially relief. There's the relief of finding your keys when you've been at the door for ten minutes at midnight in December. There's the relief when the plumber says your boiler's fine and doesn't need replacing after all, there was just a dead beetle in the pipe.

There had been a brief moment, maybe one tenth of a second, when I'd thought, *Not the lungs, but has it spread everywhere else?* Then I assured myself that to follow up 'it hasn't spread to your lungs' with 'but it is in your stomach, intestines, liver, kidneys and entire skeleton' would probably break some sort of medical code.

Dr Oikonomou continued to tell me the details of the surgery he was proposing, while I wallowed in relief, hearing little of what he said. It would be an ideal psychological test for someone applying to be an astronaut, to bring them into a room when they're not sure if they're going to live or die, reveal they will probably live and then immediately ask them to remember a series of instructions on the procedure for removing a string of dodgy lymph glands.

This is why one of the most consistent pieces of advice you're given by anyone who's been through a medical crisis is to always take someone with you when you're being given news by a consultant. The relief, dread, confusion, joy or fear of one piece of information blinds you to the instructions that follow. You're not often told two things in a row, one of which being that you *are* going to live after all, and the next that after the surgery you'll need to gargle with bicarbonate of soda three times a day.

My son and I got in the car to drive home. 'I wonder how long it will take before I get annoyed about anything again,' I said.

'Five minutes, when we're stuck in traffic,' he answered.

*

At the PET scan the following week, I was injected with radioactive dye in a recently built unit on the back of a truck outside the main building in St George's Hospital. I then had to wait an hour before being placed under the machine. The nurse said, 'Mr Steel, this scan you are having today is the Rolls-Royce of scans.' This was the moment when I was closest to weeping. This nurse was so proud – of the equipment she was associated with, of the ingenuity she was administering, of the expertise she was included in.

Thirty years ago, my situation may have been fatal, just as measles would have been a century earlier. But now it probably wouldn't be. Because physicians and doctors and scientists have dedicated themselves to blasting away these cellular mutations, because nurses and cleaners and caterers have run the hospitals, having arrived from all over the world, because campaigners and writers and trade unionists created a health service and defended it from those who try to undermine it.

As well as this, there is nothing like cancer to make you feel the depth of warmth around you. I was only at the start of this process but already my son, daughter and so many friends had taken me to appointments, listened to my complaints, lived each moment, taken the piss, told me they couldn't wait for my voice to not work for a few months, talked about cricket and been utterly fucking magnificent in every way and I adored them all even more than I had before.

During the hour of waiting for the dye to run through me, I was placed in a delicate room with flowers painted on the walls. There was a television if I fancied it, but I made a couple of calls about a leak in the bathroom, then sat under this extraordinary machine that would analyse my cells and locate the precise contours of this poxy tumour.

The results of that scan confirmed that the cancer hadn't spread past its second site, the first of which was probably in a lump in my throat, which they would take out during an operation. Now the parts that Dr Oikonomou had told me that I hadn't been able to hear would have to be endured. After the operation, they would prepare me for radiotherapy and chemotherapy, like a chicken being seasoned before being placed into an oven.

While some parts of me, such as my teeth, would still be governed by St George's at Tooting, this next stage of treatment would take place at University College Hospital in central London.

I had a curable cancer, but it was still cancer. I felt like there was a leopard in my house, locked in a room. I'd contacted the leopard authorities and they assured me they were used to dealing with leopards like this, and they had a plan for removing the leopard, though it would take a while, and two or three times a day I could still hear it growl. I was relieved as much as could be possible, but even so, at odd moments I'd think, *Oh my god, there's a fucking leopard in my house.*

Three

I Need a Doctor

I'd only been under general anaesthetic once before, to have an ingrowing toenail removed when I was 20. I have a vague memory of declaring my love for the nurse as I was going under and, a few hours after the procedure, calling a mate to pick me up so I could get to the pub.

Would this be similar?

The reason for the operation was the scans hadn't revealed the location of my 'primary' cancer. This was the sort of phrase I'd heard, vaguely, when other people's cancers were discussed or when a doctor on a TV drama was urgently rattling through a series of medical phrases to make the show seem authentic.

But now I had to learn what it meant. All cancer starts from one source, one group of cells that reproduce in an unhealthy way, and this process can spread to all sorts of areas which will all have to be dealt with, but the primary has to be found. It's the little bastard from which all other problems arise, the chief villain in its hideout like the maniac in a James Bond film. All the minions, the Oddjobs and the hulks with razor teeth can be destroyed, but there can be no lasting peace until that primary little fucker is eliminated.

The tumour in my neck, firm and lumpy and obvious, was a secondary cancer. But where was this primary, that was smart enough to evade detection by even the Rolls-Royce of scans? There was a lump under my tongue heading into the throat, and the consultants believed this was probably where it was hiding. The lump would be removed and so would my tonsils and they would all be analysed. Then they could plan to get rid of it and to zap out the secondary cancer with radiotherapy and chemotherapy.

That sort of made sense. It didn't sound that bad. People have surgery all the time, then they're back at work in a couple of days, like I was after the toenail. I remember the consultant telling me that my throat would be extremely sore but they would give me lots of painkillers, that I'd find it hard to swallow, I'd be exhausted and my voice would change for a while and I'd be useless for some amount of time but it was hard to say how much and that if I found any blood in my throat after the operation, I had to get to the hospital quickly as that could be disastrous. I interpreted this as *I'm sure it won't be too bad.*

As with any worrying episode that looms before you, it hovers as a vague unease, then solidifies into a knot of anxiety in the stomach, which feels like it's being twisted by a corkscrew, when you're given a date when it will take place. Suddenly there's a definite number of hours before it all happens, so I was told that on 9 October, I would report to the section of the hospital where they do the operations, and later that morning Dr Oikonomou and some people I'd never met would reach inside my anatomy and cut bits out of it.

My mind must have concluded that they said this would happen at some point, but they'll probably never get round to it – you know what people are like. But now the forms had been completed and the bed had been booked; the insurance documents had been emailed and someone was compiling a list of the instruments they would use to saw chunks off me.

What made it easier to contemplate was the wonderfully satisfying lack of choice.

This sensation arose repeatedly, and it's a blessing, because when there's no room to ponder if there's a possible way to get out of something, you have to accept it. The only way to wriggle out of whatever treatment they offered was to let the cancer spread, and die.

I became familiar with this sense of surrender. I'd be told what they were going to do, allow myself a tenth of a second to consider how unpleasant this might be, then ask them to get on with it.

You can challenge the details and the timing, possibly the method, and ask for a second opinion, but the fundamental issue is settled already. To complain that you don't want to go through whatever they suggest because it will be horribly unpleasant is like arguing with a fire as it rampages through your house. You can yell, 'I can't abandon my vinyl collection, I've spent all my life putting that together' at the flames, but by then your records will be ablaze anyway and now you've wasted time instead of running down the stairs.

Maybe this is why I didn't investigate very closely the mechanics of this operation. I would let them cut out the bits they said they needed to cut, then move on to the next task.

Even so, this would be the first actual physical way I'd been affected by this cancer.

Until now I'd had appointments and scans, needles and facial expressions, but now I would have an actual lump cut out, like someone with proper cancer. For a few weeks I carried on my life with alarming normality. I carried on touring my show, yelling and jumping and singing for two hours a night. I went to the pub, I went to the gym, I felt no pain or tiredness and there were moments when I wondered if there was no point in going through the trouble of this operation as I hadn't suffered at all from the cancer and maybe cancer wasn't as bad as people have made out.

But the operation wouldn't be that intrusive, I thought. People have them all the time. I rationalised it the same way I do my fear of flying. There are people who travel on planes thousands of times; it will all be done on Monday and I'll be back to normal by Thursday.

On the Sunday I drifted through the eerie normality of a day before a major event in your life. I went to a cafe; I drove across London. In the evening I played the piano and sang some silly songs, maybe because subconsciously I knew I was giving the voice a last run before it would be taken away, the way you might let a dog hump your leg one last time on the night before you have his nuts removed.

Amid the anxiety there was a hint of curious excitement. This would be a whole new adventure. No life is complete if you don't feel all the emotions, experience all the sensations. There are the obvious ones: love, travel, rejection, friendship, heartache and so on. But have you ever truly lived if you've never been arrested, never resigned from a job in a tantrum, never been stuck in a strange town with no money, never had sex up against a tree and never had a major operation?

I arrived at the hospital at 7am as instructed, where couples, whole families, people on their own in their eighties, shuffled to register at a desk.

'Name?' asked the bored, tired woman to each person in turn.

If I'd suddenly arrived there out of space and been asked where I was, I'd have assumed I was at a hotel reception. Each person gave their details and signed a form, then the receptionist gave some instructions she'd given several thousand times before: 'Take a seat opposite, you'll be called in the next few minutes, toilets are on your left, next?'

I expected her to add, 'Have you stayed with us before? Evening meals begin at seven thirty, before that you can get snacks from the cafe which is located behind the maternity ward, room service is available at all times until your anaesthetic, the lifts to the operating theatre are down the corridor and on your right.'

In front of me in the queue was a man in a tastefully crumpled jacket, arm round a blonde woman in a matching chequered suit who was trying to smile along with him. They'd acknowledged this was an important day, aware it's disrespectful to arrive for an operation looking scruffy.

They gazed at each other, her controlled concern reflecting his reassuring smile, so you knew it was him who was about to be operated on.

While there were still three people between them and the reception desk, they squeezed each other tightly. You can probably measure the gravity and uncertainty of each operation by the tightness of the squeeze that the patient and their loved ones combine in while they wait for their turn at that reception desk.

They relaxed their grip and shuffled forward. 'Name?' the bored, tired woman asked them.

When it was my turn, I filled in the form and sat on the plastic seats before a screen the width of the wall on which Sky News was reporting from Israel. I felt an unexpected breeze of relief, the moment I'd often dreaded. My major surgery had arrived, and it didn't feel so bad.

My name was called and I went into a tiny room to change into the classic hospital backless gown and remove my trousers in exchange for surgical socks, the thick, tight, thigh-length leggings that may serve some medical purpose or may be to ensure there's no chance of you running off in a panicked bid to escape.

I re-entered the waiting room, the first to emerge, and walked across the floor saying, 'Next we have Mark, modelling the autumn season's backless NHS gown and surgical stockings, designed by Coco Chanel and already massively popular in Milan.' A couple of the other patients giggled, which ignited a few others to join in.

At last, my cancer was getting laughs. And at 8.15 on a Monday morning. I was enjoying this.

Then an assortment of hospital employees arrived to give me information. An anaesthetist explained the procedure for placing me in a temporary coma and gave me the names of the chemicals they would use, as if I was likely to say, 'Ooh, propofol and etomidate, my favourites.'

A surgeon asked if I knew what the operation was supposed to achieve and a nurse read out a series of possible catastrophes that could take place. I had to sign a form to give my consent and then I was placed on a trolley and wheeled down some corridors with someone in a gown and mask on each corner.

This seemed unnecessary. Couldn't I walk there? I'd been parading across the waiting room pretending to be a fashion model 20 minutes ago.

We reached the point where I was trolleyed into a room off this bewildering corridor, feeling slightly proud that I was allowed in, as if I had a purple VIP wristband at a rock gig.

A mask was placed over my mouth and a surgeon asked what work I did. I told her I was a comic and she said, 'Oh, what sort of clubs do you appear at?'

'I usually do shows in theatres,' I told her.

'Oh,' she said, and made it clear she had never heard of me.

I remember formulating a sentence ready to say the words 'I thought I was famous but now I realise I'm obviously not' in a jokey 'An anaesthetist has just put a mask on me but we can still enjoy a light-hearted exchange' kind of way. But I got as far as 'I thought I was famous' and passed out.

It troubles me now that those surgeons have every legitimate reason to think, *What a wanker.*

*

One of the most disconcerting experiences is knowing you were unconscious. For three hours I was operated on but somehow I wasn't aware of it. Surgeons found a piece of me and cut it out and I was oblivious to all this.

I awoke and had a vague awareness that this was a positive sign: I'd had the operation and I seemed to be alright.

I was back on the trolley, being wheeled somewhere, with someone on each corner again. What I can't explain is that I thought I was in France. I asked in French if the operation had finished, which was a stupid question in any language. I asked how long it had taken, and if it had gone well. They didn't answer; instead they looked bemused and maybe amused and I didn't think this was professional.

I asked where I was going and these faces looked down at me from four angles and still refused to engage with me, and this went on until I arrived at the critical care ward for patients fresh out of an operation, and I wondered if something had gone wrong with the procedure but they weren't telling me.

It's always slightly humbling when you have to admit that whatever you've been adamant about for the last two minutes is clearly wrong, but that's quite a bit worse when the fact that you've got wrong is you thought were in France where everyone spoke French and you were actually in St George's Hospital in Tooting.

Then it occurred to me that the surgeons were thinking, 'This twat's even more pretentious than we thought.'

I became familiar with my new surroundings; I was attached to a drip and to a tube with a button on it that would pump morphine into me if I pressed it. My other arm was clipped to a machine that measured how much oxygen I was breathing. All of these devices led to cannulas in my arm or hand that were taped and led somewhere but I couldn't work out which went where, like when you're trying to figure out which of seven tangled TV cables go into which socket.

A curtain was drawn round me and a nurse came in to take my blood pressure, adding that she'd seen a report in the *Sun* that I'd got cancer. Occasionally a nurse cheerfully but without explanation checked a series of readings on the machines I was connected to. I learned that the oxygen reading shouldn't dip below 95, though once it dropped to 40 and made a deep beeping noise as this would mean I was gasping to death, so a nurse walked in and tapped the machine, then it went back to 95 and she left.

This seemed like a sequence of dreamy fantastical scenes that belonged in an incomprehensible arty film.

'Alright, Mark,' said the man in the bed opposite as his curtain was removed, and I recognised him immediately, although he now wore a hospital gown instead of a tastefully crumpled jacket.

The NHS was struggling to survive, he said, with all the privatisation sweeping through it. I admired his capacity to start a conversation with a stranger with a political rant a few minutes after waking up from general anaesthetic.

He'd had a few operations, he told me, and the most troubling part was the stress it put on his family. And over the following hours as we lay clipped to our respective drips, cables and machines, we talked about Israel and football and Jacob Rees-Mogg and kidney failures and tried to work out where it was he'd seen me on stage a few years ago, occasionally interrupted by the arrival of a nurse with a thermometer or a tiny plastic cup full of tablets.

This wasn't so bad, apart from the lack of mobility. And because of an article about the cancer diagnosis in a newspaper, the story had been mentioned on the news and I received about a thousand messages by text, email and social media that I read through, amazed and slightly bewildered and a tiny bit overcome by the volume and compassion oozing from them and the emotions of it all, enhanced, I expect, by the fact that my body was still crammed with a cocktail of drugs so potent they'd propelled me into a sleep so deep I didn't notice that some people were cutting into my throat.

In this dreamy state I drifted through the hours of being clipped to a hospital bed, and my unnatural state was probably supplemented by immense relief. Because however much I'd told myself there was nothing to worry about, I had been thoroughly worried and admitted to no one, including myself, how worried I was - and now I'd had the operation and whatever condition I was in, I hadn't woken up without a stomach or with a wooden tongue or any of the million things that had crossed my mind as possible outcomes.

I knew it would be tricky to sleep, but to ensure it was impossible the lights flickered and the machines beeped in perfect co-ordination, the oxygen monitor groaning and the drip complaining *nur nur nur* like a sarcastic teenager. There was also another machine that displayed figures that were never explained, and could have been my temperature or heart rate or possibly the cricket score of a game taking place in India.

But whatever it was it coughed out a high-pitched beep at random moments through the night.

Nurses arrived to take my blood pressure, carry out tests

and bring medicine, but the moment of adventure I looked forward to was when, once every two hours, I untangled myself from all the cables, did a wee into a cardboard vase, then whispered 'nurse' through the curtains. But all pleasure brings guilt and when I first did this I felt awful for disturbing this poor nurse so I could hand her a cardboard pot of wee. 'I'm really sorry,' I said, and she told me there was no need to be sorry.

The second time, I said sorry again and added, 'Next time I'll put some flowers in to make it nicer.'

I couldn't tell if she really hated my joke or if everyone makes that joke and she hated it because of its miserable unoriginality. My confidence was getting battered in the medical system.

Throughout the night I read more messages, from comics and strangers and people I'd not seen for several years; Phill Jupitus sent a cartoon strip he'd drawn in the style of *Viz* magazine called 'Steely's Tumour and Its Inappropriate Humour'.

Cancer is a marvellous way to be reacquainted with everyone you know.

To my right was a Polish man who spent the night playing clips on his iPhone. At about 4am he turned up the volume so instead of a background buzz, it was now loud enough that I could hear every Polish word, followed by his deep gurgles of laughter. I lay there pondering whether it was worth the effort to get up and ask him to turn it down. Eventually I concluded I wasn't all that busy so I should have a go. I unclipped one cable, then another, untwisted something that got caught round an ankle and eventually unhooked one leg enough that it could gently kick the curtain that separated us. 'Can you turn it down please, mate,' I asked, and he did.

I was as irritated as you can be when you're still dripping with anaesthetic, so the next morning I was pleased with the way he redeemed himself as a human being.

Because in this ward, the critical care unit for patients who have just had an operation on their cancer, he calmly took out a cigarette and started to light it.

'Noooo,' shrieked a nurse, as his expression suggested he was bemused by the fuss and wanted to say, 'In my village we smoke DURING the operation.'

Half-giggling out of disbelief, she took away his cigarette and tried to explain this was a no-smoking critical care cancer unit.

Then she led the Polish man, dragging his drip behind him, out of the ward, and they got into the lift and went downstairs, appearing outside where he could legally enjoy his cigarette. That is the sort of behaviour that earns nurses the nickname of 'angels'.

Four

Strangers in the Night

I was in the hospital for two days after the operation, which is long enough to absorb the rhythm, the range, the frustration and the overwhelming compassion of the world that flows through the building.

In the space of 20 minutes a doctor from Egypt checked inside my mouth for signs of blood from the operation, a nurse from Togo took my blood pressure, an Irish dentist checked my gums where a tooth was taken out during the operation and a white bloke of about 30 from south London gave me a box of nutrition drink from his van, saying, 'You'll need eight of these a day if your swallowing gets to be a problem. I won't lie, it tastes fucking 'orrible,' as he played his part in this global effort to keep me alive.

When I came back from the meeting about the nutrition drinks, there was a note on my bed from the man with the jacket, saying he'd been moved and he was sure I'd recover quickly and he would come and see me at a show when we were both in less need of critical care.

I was unclipped from most of my cables and moved to the less critical unit, next to a hockey player with an injury he'd sustained at the weekend, and opposite Noel, who was 75 and spoke to everyone as if he was a fruit trader in a London market in 1972.

'Alright, darling, you here to take me blood pressure? It's a wonder it's not through the roof wiv all I have to put up wiv. I'm only joking, love, here you go, that's it, how are you today? Did you get in alright, 'cos you had trouble wiv the buses yesterday, didn't you?'

When the Jamaican man arrived with the breakfast cereals on a trolley, Noel called to him: 'Sorry, Carl, I can't have nuffin' today, I've got my op in a few hours. You got a few days off after today, ain't yer? That's a relief, innit?'

He asked me what I was in for and told me he was about to go for his eleventh operation, this time for the removal of a kidney, which was the latest organ his cancer had spread to. 'You'd think it would get easier after a few but it don't seem to,' he said.

He lived with his daughter and her two sons. 'When I left the house yesterday my grandson said, "Here, Granddad, if you don't come back, can I have your bedroom?" Ha ha, bless him, you've got to laugh.'

I felt guilty about all the times I'd been crotchety or impatient because of my relatively tiddly cancer, and wasn't more like Noel, the model cancer patient, facing each tumultuous episode with a joyous sense that fear is pointless, the way it's claimed people dealt with the Blitz.

I was told my voice would be altered for a while after the operation but I didn't ask for any details. The word 'altered' left a lot of questions. 'Weakened' would have been clear, or 'croaky'– but 'altered'? Would I spend two weeks sounding like Jacob Rees-Mogg? Instead, it was a few notes deeper, slightly underwater and I couldn't pronounce the clipped part of words so I sounded like a reformed gangster on a documentary, whose voice has been changed for his protection so they can't be identified and then murdered by their old colleagues, as he says, 'They used to call me "Handyman" because I attacked people with chisels and a paintbrush.'

But this wasn't too bad, was it? I'd be home soon, with a mangled voice and instructions to rest, and then I'd be someone who'd had an operation and once it was over I was fine.

In the surreal environs of the hospital, your thoughts travel to all regions, especially at night. If I was a shark to my granddaughter, would she enjoy it all the more because of the twisted voice and be disappointed when it went back to normal? What mischievous comment would Shappi have made about my post-operation poise? At what point would she have engaged the nurses by making some sort of enquiry about carrying out colonoscopies?

I was discharged and given a box full of medication, I thanked all the staff and tapped on Noel's curtain to wish him good luck. 'Hello,' he said, quite meekly.

I put my head between a gap and saw him lying on his side, staring straight ahead. He didn't move.

'Hope it all goes well today, Noel,' I said, 'I'm sure it will. I'm off now, it was lovely to talk to you.'

But he wasn't really listening. 'I'm frightened,' he said.

I shook his hand and smiled. I hope he's alright.

*

Leaving a hospital is a bureaucratic exercise that can be more of a challenge than the operation you had.

You pack your bag, fold up the sheets, clear away the tissues and sit in anticipation, like someone eagerly awaiting the cab that will take them to the airport for a holiday.

Then you become aware that 40 minutes has passed by.

But you can't go until the doctor, who two hours ago said you could go home this morning, and that she'd be back in a minute to sign you off, comes back to sign you off. And nobody knows where she is.

They also have to fetch your medication. And when someone goes off to get something, a lot of time can pass before you see them again.

This isn't anyone's fault. You would have to be especially entitled to complain that the bloody doctor is attending to other people, and it doesn't matter that they've been called to a patient whose aorta has burst, she promised to bring my anti-sickness capsules so she should tell the other bastard to wait.

Most of the time a hospital ward has the opposite temperament to the image conveyed in the dramas. There's no sense of panic or urgency; the staff amble at the pace of a cricket umpire, not out of lethargy but as part of the sense that everything is calmly under control. So you wait and wait a while longer and you wonder what happens if the doctor who can sign your release paper has left the building and had a nervous breakdown and flown back to her family in Côte d'Ivoire, does that mean you have to stay here for three years?

Then she arrives with a document to sign and tells you she's sorry she's taken so long, but she's covering for three positions that have been unfilled for a year, so you feel guilty about being frustrated, and slightly guilty for being let out as you bid farewell to the other patients.

As I was leaving I was given a final warning that if I coughed up blood, I had to get to a hospital quickly as 'that could get exciting', and I nodded along at the warnings she had to give for legal reasons, and with that I was free to go.

I'd done it. I'd had an operation and a lump removed along with my tonsils and I felt fine, although that may have been connected to my body being full of anaesthetic and a little bit of morphine. The surgeons had played their part, I suppose, but I could be proud of my achievement.

Now I could recover for a few days and have it confirmed that the primary cancer had been in the lump and then begin the treatment to get rid of the tumour and be cured.

Within two days I was eating ice cream and watching cricket with my friend Matthew, who lives nearby. Matthew was a perfect companion, one of the few people as obsessed with watching sport as I was, but he was also a hypochondriac, which made him an ideal person to watch cricket with two days after an operation.

Matthew used to write a weekly column in the *Guardian* called 'Diary of a Hypochondriac'. Each week he would list a series of illnesses he was sure he was suffering from, giving us details such as 'My bowels are not so much irritable as dangerously psychotic.'

One of the qualities of a hypochondriac that I'd never appreciated before I knew him, is that they are astonishingly knowledgeable about every aspect of the human body. So he regularly made observations that sounded to me like 'The oxydidrafabimant tablets they've given you should ensure there's no capillarific inflammation of your tibularities'.

Matthew left and I went to bed, but I woke up in the middle of the night, coughing. No one had mentioned I might cough this much, but untroubled I walked to the bathroom and coughed some spit into the sink.

Still half asleep, I looked at the spit and I can remember the moment, maybe a third of a second, when I was working out what sort of spit it was. Because it was blood. It took the whole of that moment to compute it was blood, because it was so unexpected. Just as if you went to the toilet, looked down before flushing and saw that you'd pooed out a whole fresh cucumber, I didn't understand what was in the sink.

It was definitely blood. I spat again, because it was possible maybe that the blood was left over from the day before. There was more blood. I went downstairs and had to cough again, so I spat out some more spoonfuls of blood into the kitchen sink. I was aware that things could get exciting, so I grabbed the first clothes I could find, which were the clothes I usually go on stage with, including a pair of slightly sparkly shoes, went outside into the rain and called Matthew. 'I need to go to A & E,' I said through the pond of blood in my mouth, which I spat onto the pavement.

I started to feel dizzy and wondered what this looked like to anyone watching through a bedroom window from over the road. My two contending thoughts were a) I might be dying and b) I hope the people opposite aren't saying, 'You'd think he'd spit up blood inside the house.'

Several months later, he told me he'd had a huge spliff just before I called, so he arrived in a cab and when we got to A & E the conversation at reception went something like:

RECEPTIONIST: Can I take your name, please?

ME: Ungx blood ungng

MATTHEW: Um right, hang on, yes, he had an operation, and he's coughed up blood, I think it's his arterial palindrome reflux.

The receptionist made a note and we walked to join the lines of disconsolate people, who were holding the parts of them causing acute pain.

I'd walked three paces when my name was called. This was marvellous because I'd avoided the hours of gazing into a nocturnal trance that you expect at A & E. But it was terrible because my condition was one that made the medical experts shriek, 'Fuck all these other people waiting, this bloke needs to be slapped onto a bed and have things stuck into him NOW.'

I was slapped immediately onto a bed and a doctor asked me a series of questions while he examined my notes.

I indicated that it was difficult to speak, so Matthew answered on my behalf, with phrases such as 'A recent otorhinolaryngological procedure has produced haemorrhaging from the pharynx.'

'Are you a doctor?' he asked Matthew.

'No, I'm a hypochondriac,' he answered.

This was the conversation I was listening to as I lay in the emergency room, having been considered more of an emergency than all the people in the building called 'accident and emergency'.

The ear, nose and throat specialist arrived, a spirited, slightly camp soul called Mike with an accent I guessed as mid-Scotland. He held a light to my mouth and looked inside, poking under my tongue and searching, I presumed, for anything that might be disastrous.

After a few minutes, in which I'd been pondering if this was my last night alive, he said, 'Right, Mr Steel,' with slightly camp authority, then looked directly into my eyes from two feet and said, 'The first thing I need to say to you is very important - I LOVE your shoes.'

And in that moment I knew I was alright. I'd like to vote for that as the most brilliant piece of doctoring of the year.

*

They kept me in overnight and in the morning gave me some morphine - a larger dose than I'd had before. So I sat on the bed listening to commentary of a World Cup cricket match while staring straight ahead.

I wasn't too bothered about the score but was soothed by the rhythm of the commentators, as if it was a piece of gentle jazz. A friend called, alarmed that I was back in hospital, and they asked how I was. I told them it was all a wonderfully positive experience and I loved, really LOVED all the staff here, especially Bryony, the lady who brought me a toasted sandwich.

I waited for the doctor who would tell me I could go, and sat on the bed with my bag packed, smiling at the words that told me someone had scored two more runs down to deep square leg.

I decided to leave the building and buy some flowers, to decorate the house upon my return.

I drifted up Tottenham Court Road and turned in one direction or the other, looking inside Caffè Nero and a Robert Dyas hardware shop to see if they sold flowers. I turned another corner and found a Marks and Spencer, where I found and bought a bunch that looked glorious, the colours of a Wes Anderson film.

Then I walked back to the hospital, from which I still hadn't been formally discharged. And after ten minutes of walking past the same shops four times, I felt the sense of panic that must occur in someone who has wandered out of their care home and found themselves queuing up at Burger King in their pyjamas.

I became aware that I was operating in a haze of morphine and probably shouldn't be meandering around central London with no idea about anything.

'Do you know where the hospital is?' I asked a random stranger, who may have been Japanese or a Cockney in a West Ham kit or a four-year-old child – I have no idea. I followed the instructions they probably didn't give me and found my way to the magical revolving door of the hospital entrance.

I tried to explain to a doctor what had happened but mixed up my explanation with some details of the cricket commentary. Now I wanted to be coherent but couldn't manage it, or indeed manage anything apart from a simplistic grin. I learned that you can't really fight morphine. Allowing it to send you to whatever cloud you land on is one more thing about recovering from an operation that you have to meekly accept.

Five

Hungry Heart

For a few days I watched the cricket and rugby world cups in between swallowing a colourful and aesthetically pleasing array of pills. There were painkillers and laxatives, omeprazole, prednisolone, co-amoxiclav, liquids and capsules, tablets and a huge disc-shaped thing that looked like if you frisbeed it across the room and photographed it, you could convince people it was a flying saucer. I'd be fine in a few days, and after a few days I thought I'd be fine in a few more days and a few days after that I couldn't eat or drink or take any of this medication and I started to accept I wasn't recovering as well as I'd hoped, because if you're recovering you shouldn't feel much worse every day and lie on a bed coughing for an hour until the little capsule with two 'x's in its name that you swallowed an hour ago has popped out fully intact and landed on your lap.

There was a meeting with Dr Oikonomou, who told me they had analysed the lump they carved from me and couldn't see any evidence of the primary cancer in it. So they would have to start the chemotherapy and radiotherapy without knowing where this little bastard was hiding.

Is cancer allowed to do that? A primary cancer can cause the havoc of tumours and potentially lethal mutations, then just retreat and hide? Did my cancer have an invisibility cloak like Harry Potter?

The next day I tried to drink some tap water, then sparkling water, Dr Pepper, milk, Lemsip and cough medicine. But none of it wanted to go down. I'd shut my eyes and swallow, but about a minute later it would pop back out after a violent cough or burp, as if it had gone in comfortably, seen a demon with three heads and come screaming back out.

Eventually even a single drop of water refused to go in and every breath turned into a cough. I was repelling everything whole, like a magnet pinging away the wrong end of another magnet. If I carried on getting worse, would I start popping out whole organs?

One afternoon I sat on the bed with an array of unreachable targets next to me: a glass of water, a slice of bread and marmalade, a tablet. They may as well have been a harpsichord, a hovercraft and an ox. I coughed for a minute and then coughed back to the hospital, where they tried to put me on a drip, but couldn't get a cannula into my vein.

A nurse from Cameroon arrived, who told me he was the 'cannula specialist', called for when there's a patient with an annoyingly stubborn set of veins. Over the following weeks I learned that every hospital has nurses and doctors renowned for their skill at certain tasks like that. You assume that settling a needle into a vein is something every nurse can do equally well but of course there are experts. There must be debates about who's the most accurate, like the conversations in a Western about who saw the fastest gunman in the county, one of them slowly recounting, 'Many years ago when I was at Nottingham General, there was an old nurse from China, never said a word but could thread a cannula through the eye of a needle. Word has it he could do three at once. I saw him once put a cannula into the vein of a hamster right in front of me. William Tell, we called him. Then one day he just disappeared and was never seen again.'

As I lay there, in a slightly dizzy weakness from having had no food or water for several days, while a nurse eagerly poked at my vein as an exciting challenge, a porter peered through the curtain.

'Helloooo, Mark, mate,' he bellowed, 'remember Prague?'

Twenty-three years earlier I'd been to Prague on a demonstration against the World Trade Organization, and a delegation from this hospital had gone along to it. 'That was a laugh, wasn't it,' he assured me, as the nurse told me this would probably hurt a bit.

'We're still flying the flag here, Mark. Only I heard you was here and thought I'd say hello.'

'Good to see you, mate, that was a while ago,' I said, each word stretched with a squeal as the needle poked a bit further.

'Where you off to then? I'll push you up there if you like,' he offered.

'Don't know, yet,' I squeaked.

'Be good to catch up, Mark,' he said.

'It will,' I said.

'There,' said the nurse triumphantly.

'Was your veins causing trouble?' asked the porter. 'This one will always slide it in, won't you, Joseph?' He turned back to me. 'We'll have a proper chat in a minute.'

*

I was sent for a scan and then to a ward, and the next morning I was visited by a team of doctors. You can't help but feel subservient when the doctors come round in a hospital.

You're usually lying on a bed, so you look up at the circle of them as they arrive like the village elders, and you have no idea who any of them are but they all know much more about your own body than you do. And they're in suits while you're probably in a backless gown so you're not concentrating when they describe which of your organs is on the point of disintegrating, because you're desperately rearranging the gown for fear of revealing your right buttock.

So I got dressed in anticipation of my visit from the doctors, and sat up especially straight as they approached, turning down that day's World Cup cricket commentary on the radio.

'Hi, I'm Mustafa,' said the doctor. And he explained that he'd studied my latest scan and asked if I knew anything about the epiglottis.

I said I'd never heard of it.

These moments offer an instantly life-changing drama but with none of the essential build-up you'd be granted in a film or a novel. Suddenly I was confronted with the certainty that in a few moments I would find out a) what an epiglottis is and b) why my one was fucked.

The epiglottis, Mustafa told me, is a gland that sits above the throat. All you consume passes through the epiglottis, he said. It directs food and drink into the stomach and ensures it doesn't fall into any other part of your insides, where it couldn't be digested and would get in the way of whichever organ it's landed on and cause an infection. It could also block up your airways.

A risk of my surgery was that the epiglottis could be

damaged, and in my case a hole had been made. So most of the food or drink I'd consumed since then had fallen through this hole and rattled into areas that didn't want food or drink landing on them.

I find it hard not to think of my body as a workforce in hard hats, and imagine the lungs, kidney and intestine departments sounding a siren and screaming, 'Get this cottage pie out of here!'

The way my body dealt with this situation was through constant coughing, as all these organs tried to send the unwelcome food back.

As Mustafa left, he mentioned that he'd noticed I was listening to the cricket commentary. 'England are doing very badly,' he remarked. Through my twisted voice I agreed and asked, 'Which country do you support in the World Cup?'

'England,' he said robustly, and then left, leaving me to slump even further as I'd assumed he was from 'out there somewhere' because he was called Mustafa, but of course he could be English. In the space of a few weeks I'd been diagnosed with cancer and now seemed to have been diagnosed as a racist.

*

Water was flowing into my system through the drip, so I was no longer dehydrated. But I was unable to eat so I was getting hungrier and dizzier. I watched the world from my bed, never having been so aware that every aspect of human society revolves around food.

Every day is divided into sections marked by food, even in hospital. A woman from Trinidad came round every morning with a menu, printed on card like the ones you get in a Harvester. Every day she'd ask what I wanted for lunch and dinner, then see the note above my bed and sigh, 'Aaah, nil by mouth,' then turn away. Can there be any rejection more complete than that?

Then a man from Guyana who laughed at everything would arrive with a trolley, asking everyone if they wanted a cup of tea. Twice a day I'd tell him, 'I can't have tea because–' and he'd say, 'Ooh, can't have tea, can't have tea,' and somehow laugh with compassion, and not once did I manage to explain it was because of a damaged epiglottis.

When food and drink are removed from your life, you lose the shape of the day. You don't even get hungry, you stay hungry indefinitely, so the cycle of life is in disarray. Within a couple of days you adapt to a new routine, in which there's nothing to do except lie on the bed and allow hours to drift wistfully by, so you couldn't say if it was close to 1pm or 6pm. On your little screen above the bed, three reruns of *Midsomer Murders* have floated past, a nurse bounds in to take your blood pressure and you're about to tell them someone only just did it but then realise that was four hours ago.

You wonder about going to the toilet, then drift off and half an hour has passed so you make a more determined effort, sitting on the edge of the bed for two more minutes before launching yourself off, with the motivation of someone jumping out of a plane for their first skydive.

You half-read four articles in the newspaper someone

bought you, and fall asleep until the drip you're attached to pings and whoops and attracts the attention of a nurse.

In these moments it seems inconceivable there was once a time when you went to shops and cafes and sometimes just got in a car and drove to PC World. I was in the finest of hospitals with staff that were unfeasibly attentive and patient, there was a glorious view from the thirteenth floor of a building that looked down on Tottenham Court Road, while Euston station flickered below with a million people rushing to fulfil their urgent appointments. To the south I could see the television masts of Crystal Palace, one of which stretched proudly a few yards from my house. It was a view that most would marvel at. If a restaurant was placed there it would boast of the wonderful scenes you could observe as you were choosing your starter.

Within two days of being assigned to this bed, I had no interest in any of it. If someone told me the lions had escaped from the zoo and we could watch them galloping towards Leicester Square, I'd have had to force myself to bother to look.

This is why it becomes a challenge to read. Because to take in the words and process them is to consider the outside world and how this narrative relates to it, and the outside world is somewhere I felt no connection to.

Except that, while I was lying in hospital on the drip, I looked down to see a text from Shappi's dad, which made me glow. The previous year we'd visited him in hospital, as he was wired up to a series of cables following a problem with his heart.

This astonishing soul, who had been 80 for several

years, was chaotically, frenetically overflowing with concepts and inquiry and nonsensical quips that made sense if said in an Iranian accent by a man slightly stooped, with frivolous hair decorated by a charismatic hat as he dished up the stew infused with dried limes he'd been making all afternoon, before apologising for beating everyone at chess.

He would come into the house and exclaim, 'MARK! What you think of Keir Starmer?' Which was so much more interesting than the old-fashioned 'hello'. He'd pour a whisky with such enthusiasm you'd think he'd distilled it himself, and if someone suggested he shouldn't be doing this as he had to drive home, he'd say, 'It's a shame there's a law against drinking and driving, because my car is very clever, it would know I was drunk and would be very careful.'

Sometimes the family would swirl into an intense argument in Farsi, arms jerking in all directions and statements pronounced with motivation and precision, so it seemed as if they were in conflict about a critical point of Persian history or the most effective way to oppose the ayatollah, then I'd find out they were debating the quickest route to Shepherd's Bush.

Along with Shappi's mum, he had fought the despotic rulers of their country, firstly by producing a paper for Iranians exiled to Britain. In January 2023 I travelled with him to Trafalgar Square, where he spoke with an infectious optimism that made it obvious why the regime once threatened to assassinate him, at a demonstration in support of the Woman, Life, Freedom movement that had erupted to threaten the Islamic Revolutionary Guards.

Now I was following his words as I sat unable to swallow on a drip on the 13th floor of the hospital, from where it felt I could almost touch the top of Nelson's Column, under which he'd been waving his arms so defiantly that day.

He wrote that these days they can get rid of cancer, as had happened with several of their friends, with such nonchalance it made me wonder why I'd made such a fuss about it. He hoped I wouldn't forget about them all and said that once my throat was alright I had to come round for one of his meals.

It had a similar but longer-lasting effect than the liquid morphine I'd been offered an hour earlier.

*

This circle of doctors seemed to get bigger by the day, as if the head doctor was a rapper becoming more famous with a growing entourage. One day Mike was stood behind him, so I told him I still had the shoes with me and then I wondered if that was him, or if in my food-deprived state I was imagining people from random moments in my past. In a moment I might think the consultant was my mate Robert who I used to walk to school with, so he'd look puzzled as I asked if he remembered the times when we bunked off and spent all day by the pond in Farningham Woods.

Mike and the circle of eight or nine in the entourage all nodded and smiled in a neutral fashion, as they always did, then all left together.

*

You know when you say you're really hungry because it's four in the afternoon and all you've eaten all day is a Scotch egg. I can tell you that is not the beginning of hungry. After a week of not eating, I watched the news on my little TV screen and saw these aid workers in Gaza, providing small bowls of thin soup to these poor traumatised kids, and as I watched, my instinctive thought was, *You lucky bastards. I wish I could eat one of those small bowls of thin soup.*

I tried to maintain the framework of the day as much as possible, so each morning at 7.30 I unclipped my drip from the wall, and rolled it to the shower by the toilet. I manoeuvred myself out of my gown and pushed the drip, which was still attached to my arm, to the edge of the shower, washing myself with one hand. But I often felt faint and unsteady through the effort of standing under some water, so I had to rest a couple of times by sitting on the toilet, in the way that a few weeks earlier I would have sat still in the gym for a moment after ten minutes of grunting on the bench press.

My fresh clothes were laid out on the toilet seat, so I'd get dressed and go back to my bed to collect my toothpaste, toothbrush and razor; the completion of every stage was an achievement, one of the stations along a marathon route where a volunteer passes a sponge to the runners.

It was all such a performance and so tempting not to bother after a week of hunger. I could see how people give up when they're frail or depressed and the effort to maintain yourself seems so great and the reward so apparently small. In my case, the immediate prize was that once I was dressed, I could sit on the bed and watch *Only Fools and Horses* in my clothes instead of my pyjamas.

It was a lesson in how quickly your spirits can plummet. I'd been here almost a week. How must people maintain a positive attitude when they've been in prison for three years, or are taken hostage or lost at sea? I wonder if Nelson Mandela still made the effort to clean his teeth on day 3,296 in prison.

At a test to see how fucked my swallowing mechanism was, a dietician and speech therapist decided it was completely fucked. So they recommended a feeding tube to be inserted into my nose and down to my stomach.

This was a moment of unrestrained relief and solace: I was so lucky, I was going to have a piece of plastic inserted into me, quite uncomfortably I was warned. But then I could squirt a specially designed nutritional liquid through the tube so I could once again become strong enough to have a shower without needing to stop and rest halfway through.

Before I'd been so dependent on the health system, I assumed every part of a modern medical procedure involved 3-D digital models of your nervous system and microscopic fibres illuminating your intestines.

But one magical aspect of modern health is that alongside these amazing innovations, it can be so endearingly beautifully basic.

A nurse from Cork arrived at my bed with a length of hollow yellow plastic and a pair of scissors. She held it up, said, 'That should be enough,' and cut the plastic so it was about three feet long.

She looked like a presenter from *Blue Peter* in 1973, about to show us how to make a bubble machine out of a piece of plastic and a ping-pong ball.

Then she asked which nostril I preferred, and stuck the tube up it. It turned the corner towards my throat and began its descent. But there's a narrow part of the throat and as the tube rattles through that, every fibre and instinct within you wants to close the throat and scream. So I closed my throat and screamed and the tube was pulled away.

I tried again, slightly motivated by the consequences of failing to get this tube into my stomach including starvation.

But the throat, in dispute with the stomach, refused to go along with it.

So they sent for Mike, who was known as the the expert. Apparently there's a method of breathing that makes this task possible. You have to reach a level of calm, breathing slowly and gently expelling any sense of panic. When it hits the tricky part in your throat, you hold your breath for a few seconds and swallow hard. In that moment, Mike lowered the tube, reassuringly exclaiming, 'That's lovely, now let's do that again.'

During these moments I could hear actual voices in my head. It wasn't a conversation, it was two voices speaking at once, one unemotional, assured, wisely repeating that my body and mind were at one, and if I remained at peace the tube would soon be in place and I could start to take in nutrition. The other was shrieking, 'There's a length of plastic bought from a hardware shop being forced into my throat, get the fucker out NOW!'

The calm voice didn't even answer the loud one, so I did as Mike asked, until my calm voice said, 'I'm like a

Tibetan fucking monk here,' and a few more times Mike said, 'That's lovely, we're well on the way,' until I could delight in having a yellow tube reaching from my stomach out through my nose and dangling in front of me, so I looked like a surrealist piece of art called 'the Elephant'.

I could feel it, rattling against the inside of my throat where nothing ought to rattle.

'Does that feel alright?' asked Mike.

'It's very uncomfortable,' I said, 'I can feel something stuck in the back of my throat.'

'Ah, there's a reason for that,' he said. 'It's because you've got a length of plastic stuck in the back of your throat.'

I was hoping he'd tell me that my shirt clashed terribly with the bedsheets but he had to attend to someone else.

*

Shappi continued to send me messages, which I could not – dared not – read. I couldn't even contemplate sorting out the branches of my apple tree, which my neighbour had tactfully suggested I trim back out of his yard, so there was no space in my mind for addressing a ruptured love affair. There were times when I struggled to think beyond, *I hope I'm still alive for next summer's Olympics* and *Where is the liquid for the nebuliser?*

If the thoughts I was finally able to tap into, during brief moments of peace, were *She says I was obstinate but* she *was the obstinate one*, I'd have laid flat on my back in the hope the coughing started again. It would feel like being in two dramas at once, such as *Eastenders* and *Jurassic Park*. 'Not only have I got Bianca giving me earache, now there's a velociraptor in my kitchen.'

And if she'd written anything loving, I'd wish I could stroke her hair while she did her perfect impression of her neighbour who writes an itinerary for a walk to the park, and then I'd be in a right pickle.

If I'd known for certain that her messages were full of kindness, affection and understanding I would have read them over and over, like a soldier in a Belgian trench that's received a letter from his love back home.

Twice I got as far as composing a message to send to her, before changing my mind as I felt I had a house full of problems that I was just about coping with mentally, and if another one was tossed into it, it would be like having a leopard *and* a rhino in the house and the floorboards would collapse.

*

Once the tube was fitted into my nose, I could pour the nutrition drink into a cup and suck it into a syringe, then attach it to my new appendage and push it through the tube into my stomach. Three months earlier I would have found the thought of this hideous and tragic, but I was deliriously relieved with every shove of the syringe.

Three days later I left the hospital, occasionally noticing a surreptitious glance from someone as they walked past, unable to resist looking to see what the yellow object was that was dangling from inside my nose.

Two weeks later I was awarded a PEG, an identical tube but it's inserted directly into the stomach.* This involves a minor operation, for which I was sat in a room and for legal reasons I was warned about what could go wrong. A camera would be lowered into my stomach, so the surgeon could see where to direct the tube through a piercing that would be similar to the one made for an earring.

The camera could catch on something and scratch it or infect it or ruin it and there were so many possibilities that I drifted off, and he might as well have been saying 'there's a 1 in 50,000 chance that the tube gets wrapped round your liver and pulls it out of your ear,' or 'there's a 1 in 400,000 chance of an allergic reaction to the tube that causes you to believe you're Helena Bonham-Carter,' or 'it could broadcast film of your digestive system directly onto BBC One'.

Then a mild sedative sent me into a trance until I looked down to see a tube protruding from my stomach instead of from my nose, which was altogether more satisfying.

From then on I would squirt ten bottles of the nutrition drink a day into that tube, along with eight litres of water and a variety of medicines. It seems peculiar that you can't taste anything as it goes in, though it shouldn't seem odd as you've bypassed everything that can taste.

So the business of feeding yourself becomes entirely functional; all pleasure is removed.

I suppose you could pretend you were preparing a meal by pouring the liquid into a bowl and sprinkling a pinch of paprika onto it.

* PEG stands for percutaneous endoscopic gastrostomy.

But all changes to your body are relative and this stomach tube was a little treasure that I looked at with warmth, the way other people would admire a new piano or set of golf clubs.

One problem I hadn't anticipated was that if someone visited me at home, I'd feed myself through the tube, but feel awkward as I was feeding myself without offering anything to my guest. My instinct was to say, 'Would you like some? I've got plenty spare. I'll have to carry out a medical procedure but it's no trouble.'

One friend who came round told me that he'd seen one of these stomach tubes before, on a man who drank every night in the Crystal Palace Wetherspoons. 'Every evening,' he said, 'he would syringe some beer from a glass, attach it to the tube and pump it directly into his stomach. Then when he'd done a whole pint, he'd squirt a glass of whisky in as a chaser.'

Six

The Mask

I'd never heard of radiotherapy. A friend asked if that was where I was locked in a room listening to Chris Moyles's morning show until I screamed, 'Alright, I'm cured!' Some patients may be given that, but I had the more typical version, which is a series of blasts of radiation, targeted precisely at the area of the cancerous tumour. The rays are strong enough to kill the cells they're aimed at.

So the team that's ascribed to your treatment calculates precisely where the mischievous cells are, through a series of scans. Then they create a mask for your head.

This is made out of a tough plastic which is moulded around you in a special session, like the ones you hear an actor has to go through each morning in make-up before playing an ogre with the head of a dragon. I lay on a bench while the soft warm substance was squashed around me to form the exact shape of my head. Then it hardened into a fierce shield, like the mask of a Japanese Kendo warrior, except it extended to the neck and shoulders. This would lock me in place during the treatment, in which I would be bolted onto a bench so a particle accelerator could fire the radiation into the tumour.

After the mould had been made, the team tested it on me by pushing it as firmly as possible onto my face, so I could feel it pressing onto me, so tight that there wasn't room to close my eyes. Then they said, 'Now we're going to bolt it down.' What? This wasn't tight enough?

All of this is to ensure the rays are fired exactly into

the cancerous area; they have to be much more accurate than someone washing their car with a jet wash.

I heard the *clump clump* of a series of bolts pushing into their slots and the hardened mask clasped around my contours so that for a moment I thought, *I can't put up with this.*

But then, as with every other part of the process, you immediately reconsider and think, *I HAVE to put up with this.*

Like a soldier that knows they'll be shot for desertion, the problems you'll face by going into battle are much less than the problems you'll face by lining up in front of a firing squad.

You hear the radiotherapist tell you calmly that you'll be locked in for about ten minutes, then they count down each minute until they tell you, 'We're leaving the room now to watch the screen.'

That induces the next irrational moment of panic as you think, *What if they just leave me here?*

You know this isn't likely. You know there would be serious consequences if the entire radiotherapy team bolted a patient rigidly through a mask onto a bench, then left the hospital for several hours to go shopping.

*

One week later I entered the basement of the hospital for my first dose of radiation.

'Mark, could you change into your gown, please,' said the calm youthful machine operator, with the diffident, matter-of-fact, slightly bored air of an aeroplane captain telling everyone to return to their seats and put their seatbelts on.

As I put on the flimsy but highly unsexual gown, I could hear the machine whirring over the previous patient. Eventually there was a series of serious beeps, the sort you get in a science fiction film warning everyone in London about incoming spaceships. A neon light flashed the words DO NOT ENTER.

I couldn't help but wonder how calamitous it would be if you ignored all the warnings and walked in. Maybe you'd tear a hole in space and time and find yourself in the First World War.

A couple of minutes later the patient emerged. They seemed alright, though it's possible this bald man of about 70 was only 15 when he'd gone in there a few moments earlier. 'Good morning,' said the cheerful nurse as I took my turn, as if they were about to paint my nails.

'Can you just lie on the bench for me?'

The machine was a looming matrix of plastic and glass, with several arms and a separate screen to one side. At the moulding session I'd asked what that was for, expecting it to be an additional laser that fired extra radiation from a distance like a cowboy in a Western practising his shooting in the desert.

'That has Spotify on it,' they told me, 'so you can have music during the treatment if you like.'

This was wonderful. So before my first session I asked for *Favourite Worst Nightmare*, the Arctic Monkeys' second album. Anything with regular tracks would be ideal, so I could measure my ten minutes of encasement through three and a bit songs that I could pick out over the industrial clanking of my master.

Then began the routine that I became endearingly familiar with. The radiotherapist and nurse adjusted me on the bench, like a golfer carefully placing their ball on the tee.

The mask was squashed on and the bolts applied. They said a series of numbers: '1.5 right upwards of 0.6 lower left'. Then they told me they were leaving the room and I'd hear them depart, and the machine began to whirr. A grumble from the left, a click from the right, a weary resigned bleat above as it changed position, then an abrupt shudder of the bench like a tiny earthquake. By this point we were towards the end of 'Teddy Picker', the second track on the album.

Then came the siren I'd heard from outside. This was when, on certain days, my imagination got the better of me and I wondered if the radiation would go wrong and when I got up I'd have the bottom half of a chimpanzee.

Throughout this there was not the slightest sense of anything being done to my body: there's no warm glow as the radiation pours into you.

Shortly after the beeping stopped, during the early stages of 'Balaclava' (the fourth track), I heard footsteps and a voice saying, 'That's it, Mark, first one done, only twenty-nine to go.'

I was used to it already. The claustrophobia of the mask had waned, the irrational concerns were dismissed. When I described the process to other people, sometimes they'd say, 'I couldn't put up with that.'

But they could. Because however uncomfortable it may be to get bolted onto a bench in a tight hard-plastic mask, it's not as uncomfortable as leaving cancer to spread all over you and destroy your organs until you die.

'See you tomorrow,' said the radiotherapist chirpily, so I put my shirt back on and walked up the stairs onto the street as if I was perfectly normal and not at all fizzing with radiation.

*

The Suede album *Dog Man Star* was ideal to accompany radiotherapy, as was *The Greatest Hits of Dusty Springfield*, though I'm not sure whether, as Burt Bacharach produced these songs, he intended them to be enhanced by a machine growling *hynnngggg* KAKAKAKA as it approached the listener to fire radiation into their neck.

On the fourth day I skipped with an optimism I knew was misplaced. I'd had three doses and still felt lively and fancied *Red Roses for Me*, the first Pogues album, which splatters from the start like a Celtic Gatling gun. The opening track, 'Transmetropolitan', explodes with Shane MacGowan celebrating drunkenness and debauchery, which seemed appropriate for a building dedicated to health.

The mournful old prison song 'The Auld Triangle' had to battle with the fervent siren of the most radioactive moments, then I was unbolted to the line, 'Jingle bloody jangle', and I was as grateful to Shane as I have been since first hearing this magnificent racket in 1984.

I walked out onto Tottenham Court Road, four sessions done, and turned my phone back on. Shane MacGowan, it told me, iconic front man of the Pogues, had died that morning.

I don't think I've ever felt so spiritual.

The downside was that I also started to feel worse. I had been able to eat and drink again as the epiglottis slowly repaired, but I still had the tube in my stomach because the treatment would soon make it impossible again. And in a fascinating twist, as the radiotherapy burns into the cancerous area of a neck cancer patient, it damages the intricate mechanisms that are in the way. One of them is the group of cells we know as tastebuds.

They had warned me my tastebuds would be affected but I didn't expect that everything would taste of wet salt, on every area of the tongue, as if a lawn of wet salt had been carefully laid in my mouth by a very thorough gardener.

If I'd gone to a Michelin-starred restaurant where a chef had dedicated himself to making one special meal just for me, at which he'd worked tirelessly for three days, effusing about the basil he'd selected personally and the beef he'd travelled to France to procure, I could have put any component of the dish onto my tongue and squealed, 'Fuck that, it tastes like wet salt, mate, you need to sort that out.'

It wasn't just that everything tasted of wet salt. *Nothing* tasted of wet salt as well. So there was no escape.

One Monday, by a wonderful coincidence, my chemo was on the same day that my old friend Pat had the last of his post-cancer scans, completing his five years, so we met up in the canteen to celebrate. It seemed rude not to toast his final scan with anything, when I saw a bottle of an Innocent fruit drink and was attracted by its pastel pink shade, oozing health and peace and achievement and berries.

'That should rid me of this taste of wet salt,' I said to Pat. Excitedly, I poured the first sticky pink splurge onto my tongue, spat it straight back out into a paper cup and coughed. 'Ugh, it tastes like wet salt.'

It's not even the wet-salt experience of swallowing sea water, because that includes water, which offers a sense of hope that once the water has been spat out the wet-salt taste will dissipate soon after. This is wet salt that has unpacked its bags and settled in.

I played the first five Pogues albums on a loop for the rest of the day and hoped my choice of music for that morning's treatment hadn't influenced the universe in some way.

On the second Monday I chose the Happy Mondays, then as the symptoms started to kick in, I went for the soothing Algerian Souad Massi and, as a nod to the future, the young English rapper Little Simz.

By the third week the radiotherapists, one about 30 and usually an assistant of about 24, seemed genuinely eager as they asked, 'What music have we got today?' Sometimes I'd surprise them with something obscure like Eivør Pálsdóttir, the Faroese folk singer, but usually it would be something they knew such as Bowie or Eminem.

By the end of week four my voice had gone and I had to type in the album name myself before clambering onto the bench.

On the Monday of week five I typed in, very deliberately, 'Dexter Gordon, Our Man in Paris.'

*

How should you discuss your cancer? People ask you how you are, when they know you've got cancer, and it's hard not to say, 'I'm fine – apart from the cancer.'

Even the hospital staff ask that. 'Hello, how are you today?' says an effervescent nurse with an infectious breezy skip in the words, and it seems so unkind to reply that while you're managing as best as you can, the reason you're in their little room about to have your blood tested is you've got sodding cancer.

I did an interview for a national newspaper, about two weeks into my treatment, in which a journalist sat in my living room and we discussed the illness and the mucus, the hopes and the lost biopsy. Alongside her was a photographer, a cheery, sympathetic soul, and for an hour and a half the three of us talked about the side-effects, the fading voice, the coughing, the tiredness and the sickness that must have been obvious as I sat there displaying it all. Then the photographer said he'd seen me doing a show a couple of times a while ago and asked, 'So where are you performing this weekend?' He'd been sat there with me, as I croaked and spluttered my account of being in the middle of cancer treatment.

What did he think this show would look like? 'HELLO NORWICH! *Kha kha hyeak*, thanks so much *ahaaakak*. Sorry, I've just got to gob in this cup *khaaaaakkkk ahyek* – anyone in from Bungay? *Raaaakkkkakakkk* oh fuck *rakkkkakhakh*.'

I got a message from someone who had promised to help me with some administrative tasks while I was having the treatment. At the start of January, with clearly the kindest intent, she wrote, 'I hope you got some time to relax at Christmas.'

This was endearing, as if cancer's a job, and although you don't get a whole week off like most people because it's quite punishing, surely it gives you Christmas Day and Boxing Day off before you have to have cancer again on the 27th?

If I did have to carry on having cancer at Christmas, maybe I should speak to HR or ask for double pay.

But I didn't say that because they meant well. And in the same way, someone is only being kind when they say, 'I know you're probably a bit out of action at the moment, with the chemo and the radiotherapy and the operation and the cancer, but if you are able to come to our house a week on Friday, we're having a party on a kids' bouncy castle and then we're all going bungee jumping and I just thought it might cheer you up if you want to come along.'

Seven

Happy House

The chemo room at University College Hospital (UCH) is strangely soothing, as if it was designed by a hi-tech company in California, where's there's a 'chill-out space' for the workforce to lie on a bed or play pool when they're in need of mental refreshment.

A receptionist smiles and asks you to take a seat, in a manner that makes you wonder if you're about to be interviewed for a job as the new manager. The room is long and perfectly rectangular, the size of a school sports hall, with around 20 beds and 20 large armchairs dotted irregularly around the edge by the windows. There is a large space in the middle and lots of stands for the drips, some with bags of water, chemo or other solutions attached, looking like robots from the same science fiction film that included the radiotherapy sirens.

At first it looks less like a medical room and more like a Damien Hirst installation.

You sit wherever you fancy and wait for your name to be called. But it isn't really called: a nurse wanders past the line and says quietly, 'Mark Steel? Is Mark Steel here?'

'How are you today?' they ask. I do my 'Fine, apart from the cancer' line.

Then they weigh me. 'Good,' they say, 'that's good,' and I don't know what's good.

At first I thought they meant my weight was good but they even said it when I'd lost more than I should have done.

On the first day it was so relaxed it was slightly disconcerting. Was I in a waiting room for a sauna and a massage?

Then a nurse who is allotted to you for the morning arrives to put in the cannula.

Then it gets more tricky. I'd drift into my cannula routine, choosing a song to sing in my head, telling myself that by the time I got to the end, the cannula would be inserted and the discomfort would be over.

But as the weeks passed, the veins became more resistant, like a cat that refuses to get into its box for a trip to the vet. So I would try to breathe deeply and concentrate on my song, ignoring as best as I could the abrasive needle that was supposed to glide into me effortlessly but was now digging and scratching, shifting and probing as the nurse made noises like *hnnng, phoo, tup tup* so I knew this attempt would end with an 'Oh dear, your veins are VERY small and hard.'

'So it hasn't gone in?' I'd ask, interrupting the last chorus.

'No.' They'd sigh, seeming slightly defeated.

I became used to medical people tapping my arm to raise a vein for a blood test, telling me they couldn't find one, so I'd reply, 'I'd make a terrible junkie,' which they always ignored.

Then they would often ask, 'Have you another vein?' It was said in the weary tone of someone in a shop asking 'Have you another bank card?' when your first one was declined.

'I always have this trouble,' I'd say. So they'd search round me for other veins, sometimes stopping to tap one, asking me to open and close a fist, maybe they'd say, 'Let's try this one,' I'd choose another song and the whole thing would start again. Kate was the nurse who cracked this code, discovering a vein at the back of the elbow, a secret vein that most men had, she said, that was slightly awkward to get to but the easiest to invade.

Once this secret passage had been found, I could lie or sit attached to a drip, and across the room the other cancer patients would do the same, reading or doing puzzles as if they were on a sun bed.

Sometimes I would wander slowly across the open space, pulling my drip, to bond with a fellow chemo soul.

There was Alexandra who was 80; she'd been told she was too old for certain treatments although she told me, 'I am younger than the president of United States, ha ha.'

There was a bald man who always said, 'How you doing, guvnor, how many weeks of this ol' malarky you got to have then? It's alright in here, mate, no sense in complaining. I've got nuffin' to worry about wiv chemo, I've got no bleedin' 'air to start wiv.'

And there was a leukaemia patient called Dave. My most surprising conversation was with Dave. He was 70, he told me, and had been diagnosed with an unusual brand of leukaemia. The preferred cure, he'd been told by the consultant, if the doctors felt his body was strong enough to withstand it, was arsenic.

This was delivered through a drip, in the same way the rest of us were taking in the chemo.

'So that's arsenic?' I said, wondering if he was winding me up and this would end with the East End man laughing and saying, 'He's only gone and believed he was having fuckin' arsenic.'

But it was true. The arsenic kills the unwanted cells in the same way that the poison of chemotherapy kills them.

So it must always have had this cancer-curing quality. There must have been murderers in the seventeenth century who despaired, muttering, 'With guile and most wily deceit did I apply arsenic, the most wicked poison, to Sir Bartholomew's evening meal. Yet I find not only hath it not vanquished him, it hath cured his cancer and he is restoreth to the finest health.'

During my weeks there I didn't hear one person in the chemo room raise their voice or complain or speak in any way that was negative. Everyone is calm, a nurse arrives to check your bag of chemo is flowing fluently and peruses the drip efficiently and with less of a sense of alarm than a barista cleaning a coffee machine. I'm not sure I've ever known a place so devoid of negativity. In any office, at any time, someone is grumbling – about the idiots in the other department who never reply in time or the useless new lad in the warehouse. A football ground is an arena of rage: not just semi-jokey animosity towards the opponents but hatred, actual hatred, towards fans' own players. 'You're SHIT, not fit to wear the SHIRT,' they scream, with limbs jerking randomly in all directions like a fly just after it's been zapped by fly-spray.

There's none of that in the chemo ward.

Maybe I was lucky and in other hospitals the atmosphere is more fractious. Possibly there's an enlightenment that shines on people with a serious illness so that all the usual petty complaints of life are too trivial to bother with. But most likely it's that when you're in need of chemo, or indeed arsenic, it simply doesn't help to be anxious, angry and frustrated with the day-to-day details of your environment. This isn't just a piece of Zen wisdom, it's counterproductive to be furious and negative.

There's simply no point in screaming about matters that are not just beyond your control but beyond anyone's control. If you yell, 'Why do my veins have to be so annoyingly fucking small?!!!!!' who are you raging against?

You don't have to accept the state and condition of the health service as inevitable. You don't have to shrug with abandon at the declining pay of the staff, or dismiss the growing waiting lists with a surrendered grin, because they're the result of human decisions that could be different.

But if you've got cancer, and you're in a room set up to treat you for it, your best chance of getting through this is to accept the situation and calmly undergo your part in changing it, by sitting on a bed while chemo - or arsenic - is dripped slowly into your thin and useless veins, while all around is peaceful.

As well as that, I imagined Shappi in this room, who would have had an animated conversation with the bald Cockney man, discovering that his wife had four sisters and he had an affair with a ballet dancer in his twenties, and she'd have diagnosed at least one doctor with ADHD, until I was saying, 'I think we should leave, the chemo finished an hour ago.'

Eight

Breathless

Around the end of the second week of radiotherapy the wet-salt taste becomes a minor problem, next to the new change in your body that transforms you into a creature that at times is barely human.

It's very common for the treatment to batter the glands that produce saliva, and because I had a particularly high dose it mangled them in all directions. Saliva allows us to chew food, it protects teeth, it keeps the mouth moist and when it disappears the body compensates by producing mucus instead.

That was in the pamphlet I was given about the likely side-effects of my treatment.

But what the pamphlet didn't mention was the volume of mucus.

I became a machine for producing mucus, at an industrial level, like the oil that Daniel Day-Lewis strikes in *There Will Be Blood*. It suddenly spurts up and just keeps coming. You wonder where all that oil comes from and think that surely after a day or two it will run out; it doesn't seem possible that there's an inexhaustible supply.

I imagine an ecstatic Texan in a wide hat running around in the wayward mucus and squealing 'yeeehaah' as he calculates there's enough in there to last ten generations.

The ease with which this stuff reproduces would delight managers of industry. Soviet officials would boast in an announcement over a Tannoy, 'Comrades, it is with immense pride we announce a sixty-seven per cent increase in this year's production of the people's mucus.'

Every few minutes my mouth would be full of this frothy phlegm, then someone in the room would ask me a question about what I thought of that film about Napoleon, and I'd answer 'hnnngg hanungggg owtheway, OW THE WAY' as I barged into the toilet to spit it out so the next mouthful could start to form.

And the mucus, as soon as it formed, hit my tongue and tasted of wet salt. Couldn't it at least have come in mucus flavour? With all the research that goes into cancer treatment, maybe they'll find ways of making cancerous mucus into a series of different flavours, like rum and raisin or pistachio.

During week four of my treatment the mucus supply INCREASED, which I didn't think was possible. It must have attained international investment and won contracts round the world. I was probably supplying mucus to countries that don't have their own natural supply, with a pipeline running from my sink to Holland or Argentina.

At night the output was usually at its peak, as if the night-shift mucus glands were especially dedicated. To start with I would climb out of bed and position myself over the toilet, ready to spit out the latest mouthful, but often I coughed up a frothy globular deposit, and by the time I'd turned round to go back to bed, the next one had formed, so there was no point in leaving my post.

Mucus was pouring out of me with such bewildering force, I pondered whether the weight of the mucus I'd coughed up over a day was more than my actual weight, meaning I now weighed a minus amount. One night in my sleepless state of semi-consciousness I imagined a news item in which my road was flooded with my mucus, so plucky residents had to climb out of their upstairs windows into canoes to get to the shops.

One by one the fundamentals are attacked, but each time you come to accept all this as inevitable and hopefully temporary, and tell yourself that there are still plenty of ways to be calm and enjoy yourself. I'd lost the ability to eat or drink, couldn't imagine ever feeling vaguely sexual again and then sleep came under fire.

The spitting cup I'd been using was no longer sufficient; I needed a spitting salad bowl, designed to host delicately arranged leaves of lettuce and drizzles of balsamic vinegar, but now a receptacle for streams of frothy guttural spit, each one heralded with a *gnur ugh yek* sound.

Eventually there wasn't even a sufficient gap between any of the spits and coughs to fall asleep. It was like waiting to pull out at a junction but there would never, ever be a moment when anyone would let you out, so you wait for nine hours before giving up and going home.

So I would watch films on my laptop – films I'd been meaning to watch but never got round to. I watched *The Seventh Seal* and *The Searchers*, *Night of the Living Dead*, *Sunset Boulevard* and so many classics, none of which, I imagine, were made by directors who hoped their audience would watch them after 22 hours with no sleep on a laptop on their bed while coughing constantly and missing ten seconds out of each minute as they turn their head to honk up a ball of spit into a salad bowl. The cough can go on for eight hours at a time. But it's a tease. It doesn't start out as a rumbustious roaring bellow, it begins as a thin little wheeze, a pitiful excuse of a cough, that feels like it will be dispensed with after one clear of the throat. But it's like a little thread of cotton that you try to unpick, before discovering you've unravelled an entire pullover. You try to clear the little cough and it goes on; it becomes an elongated whining rasp that won't stop until you gulp and *then* comes the guttural timpani of a cough that you can imagine being signalled by a famous eccentric conductor, his elbows now scything around him as the baton flies and he commands the cough to give it all, leaving nothing behind after setting it up with a few tinkly bars. Now there's no stopping it, *AHEEUGHRRRRAWARUMEYAYAYAYACKORWORWA.*

It feels as if the cough is alive inside you, yearning to escape like the baby monster that burst out of John Hurt's stomach in *Alien.*

All you can do is get through each moment, while keeping a thought in your mind that this will pass. Eventually there will be a window of peace in which you can sleep, and one day this will stop altogether.

During these weeks I slept for an hour or two at moments when the coughing receded, until the hooter went off in the factory and the next shift began. At random points in the day if I wasn't coughing and the mucus slowed down I would rush to bed to get in some sleep while it was possible.

*

I wasn't sick after the first two weeks of chemo, which I was proud of, as if it was a result of my own skill, something you can learn, like playing the xylophone.

The day after the first chemotherapy treatment I made a meal, with salmon and cheese sauce and a delicate array of steamed vegetables, then looked at it with utter contempt, pushing it down in the way you squash down the rubbish because you can't be bothered to take it out and fetch a new bin liner.

It was the last meal I ate for several months.

On that day a low hum developed in the bottom of my stomach, and sulked in its corner like a miserable lodger. I didn't see it much but it was always there, in its own room, unsettled and unsettling, contributing nothing, so I could never forget it.

For most of the next four weeks I was in this constant state of being almost sick, until I wondered if that was worse than actually being sick.

I've always done anything I can to prevent actually being sick, even if being sick would remedy the problem by getting rid of the muck that's making me feel sick. Because I was brought up in a world in which being sick was a sign of failure. The kid at school who was sick was sniggered at, a subject of pity as a caretaker arrived with a tragic bucket of sand. Once I was 16, if you were sick after a drinking session, that was a sign of terrible effeminacy: you had proved you were untrustworthy in battle.

On a boat the real man is never sick, even in a hurricane.

All this was deep in my psyche as I stood before the toilet on Christmas Day, firing out spheres of mucus, each one queuing up to be shot out, like kids on a midsummer's day at an amusement park, being clicked into place on the log flume and hurtled down the chute only two seconds after the ones before have set off. Eventually my body couldn't sustain an assault at this rate. I felt the familiar gaseous rumble that told me I was going to be sick and that there was nothing I could do; then came the violent jerking defeat of Nutricia Fortisip 2.okcal drink launching itself up my body like a firework. You're not supposed to taste this stuff; it's just filling you with nutrients to keep you alive. But you taste it when it comes back up. Fuck my old boots, it's horrible. It's light brown and sickly without being sugary, as thick as a custard that didn't turn out to be properly thick, with a slightly sweet aroma that would normally make you think something is maliciously poisonous.

Vomiting is not just a physical discomfort, it's psychologically disturbing because you have to accept a loss of control of your own body. Once the torpedo of sick is launched from the core of the stomach, you're at the mercy of forces way beyond you.

You can try and direct it, so you don't ruin trousers, carpets and plants, but you have to surrender to it. For however long it lasts you will be sick's bitch. And chemotherapy sick has a special stamina. It doesn't simply demand the offending poison is expelled until you can return to a period of calm. You will be sick and then more violently sick and then go back to feeling sick and a couple of days later you'll have another chemotherapy session so more of the poison that was making you sick is pumped directly into your veins. It's as if you had a wretched night of vomiting from food poisoning, then two days later had to eat another plate of the same out-of-date mouldy fish that caused the trouble in the first place. So on Christmas afternoon, around the time of the broadcast of the King's speech, I stood and sat and kneeled in turn over the toilet bowl, making those desperate noises: at first an almost defiant AYEEUUUURGHH, but 40 minutes later a resigned *oh oh hnnnn wur*, which translated from sick language means, 'I give up, I'll do whatever you want.'

On and on it went, and all I could think about was being sick, and that eventually it must stop as no one is sick for ever, and a couple of times it occurred to me that it was Christmas Day.

I felt dimly aware of Christmas but it felt like a festival that other people participated in. It was like being in a small Spanish town as they have their biggest day of the year, a celebration of a saint you've never heard of, and a procession in which everyone dresses as a llama. I enjoyed watching other people rushing round shops but felt it was nothing to do with me.

But for a few days my body eased off from the worst of the afflictions. I bought a three-foot Christmas tree and a few presents and had a haircut. This was a moment of immense pride. I had a haircut! During my fourth week of chemotherapy! How hard must my hair be? Not only had it not fallen out, it needed to be cut! My hair was saying to the chemo, 'Is that all you've got?'

*

You can often underestimate the significance of an event that may seem routine to you, but to someone else is a glorious day of life-affirming sanctity. A few months earlier

I'd spent a day with someone I rarely see, who has two young sons. We went to the pub and then for a kebab, chortling through this blokey nod to the 1970s as a form of entertainment.

Several weeks later he told me that day had been momentous for him, as it was the first time he'd been out like that all day for a year. When someone is deprived of socialising and of culture, because they're constantly looking after small children or elderly parents, or due to poverty or illness, an afternoon in a cafe with a mate can be enough to revive them, to reconnect them with a part of themselves that was disappearing.

I'd only had three weeks of feeling outside of my normal world, but the amble round some shops and 15 minutes of semi-chat with Cecile who cut my hair, before my voice gave up and I fell asleep as she did the fringe, was as exciting as a trip to Disneyland for a seven-year-old.

*

By week five of the treatment I was being assaulted from all angles. The painkiller constipates you, so you're given a laxative, but it didn't make everything normal; it meant I could have a shit but painfully. We're all familiar with this situation: the dry scratching of the turd that scrapes out as if there's an angry miniature swordsman in it, lashing out in every direction.

But however painful, if you're experiencing this during week five of your cancer treatment, it's almost welcome as a change from the routine discomfort of the mucus.

Somehow the body increases the amount of mucus being produced, even though you were already at the peak of maximum possible mucus flow, according to the laws of physics. It's like discovering there's something that travels faster than the speed of light.

Every few minutes there would be a surge, bubbling from deep inside the stomach, then an intense but very brief rumble and then whoosh, out would pop a perfectly formed Cadbury Mini Egg-sized ball of mucus straight into the sink, where it would sit like a newborn kitten, slightly pleased with itself and wondering what to do next.

Even through the self-disgust and discomfort of this act – in the middle of the thoughts of *What on earth have I become?* – a bit of me would be fascinated and slightly proud.

This wasn't a sticky cumbersome dribble of mucus, the sort that amateurs cough up. It was pure and whole, and I'd admire it for a second as if I was a renowned potter and a beautifully glazed vase had popped serenely from my kiln.

By now my appetite was so suppressed that not only did I have no desire to eat or drink, I found the whole idea of eating or drinking disgusting. I watched other people eat in the way you watch a wildlife documentary in which a bird produces sick and pours it into the mouths of their young. It was as if I was observing a lesser species that hadn't advanced to the stomach PEG and still did that revolting thing where they put food in their mouth.

Before, when my swallowing mechanism was damaged, I'd been longing to be able to eat properly. I dreamed of that stew, or poached egg on toast. But now I gazed upon the Christmas dinners I would once have worshipped and saw it as a heap of debris, as inviting as a stagnant pond with a dead crow floating in it.

During the fifth week of treatment, my voice withered hour by hour, becoming fainter in the way a local radio station gradually vanishes as you drive out of range and into a different region.

For a few days I could whisper, then that went as well, so I could make no meaningful sounds at all.

Being voiceless is a confusing state and I often forgot it had gone. I'd start to sing along to whichever song was in my head, and for a moment I'd be thrown because nothing came out.

But it was more confusing for everyone else. I would mime to someone that my voice had gone, and usually they'd respond by asking how long it would be before it would come back.

So I would stand there silently, and the other person would look bemused, as if they were thinking, *Well, it's a simple question, there's no need to be rude and not answer.*

A few times I was called by someone from the hospital. This was the only time I answered the phone during these weeks, and it would be with a misty 'hawoo': an attempt to make a word out of a breath, like someone making an old-fashioned obscene phone call.

Someone from the company that delivered the nutrition drinks called one morning. A voice asked, 'Hello, is that Mr Steel? I wonder if you can tell me if it's alright to make our next delivery on Tuesday and how many bottles you require?'

I summoned up a puff of breath and tried to say, 'I can't talk,' but all I could say was an almost silent 'ekentak'.

'Did you say you can't talk?' asked the woman who could talk.

'S,' I hissed, which in my language was 'yes'.

'I'm just wondering how many bottles you need for your delivery on Tuesday?'

'Ehehe,' I breathed, as I couldn't manage 'ekentak' a second time.

'Oh right,' she said, 'well, can you tell me how many bottles you need and if it's alright to bring them on Tuesday?'

Now I was reduced to 'eh'.

Then she started saying the words slowly and loudly, as if she was an English tourist talking to an Italian: 'I SAID "HOW MANY BOTTLES?" You know, BOTTLES? HOW MANY?'

'Ofafasak,' I breathed, which in my head was 'oh for fuck's sake', and I'm now glad that can't have been intelligible. Then I turned the phone off.

I suppose she turned to a colleague and said, 'What a rude man! I asked him a simple question and just because he can't talk he didn't answer.'

Having no voice sends many people that you meet into blubbering confusion. At the hospital chemist I arrived at the counter for that week's medication. 'Can I have your name and date of birth?' asked the woman behind the counter.

So I wrote it on a sheet of paper and handed it to her. She wrote underneath, 'Have you had this medication before?'

I wrote, '<u>You</u> can speak to me,' and handed it back.

So she said hesitantly, 'Have you had this medication before?' as if she was saying her first sentence in a foreign language, which she'd learned from a phrasebook. I pondered this all the way home. Did she think, *How can he understand me when he can't speak?*

Or maybe she wrote the question as part of a scheme to show empathy with the patients, by adopting the same affliction as theirs. If someone arrives with one leg, they have to hop to the shelves and back to fetch the tablets.

My daughter accompanied me to my chemotherapy in week five of my treatment, just after Christmas. She held my hand during the 'Oh, what IS the matter with your veins?' part of the cannula process.

I'd taken a whiteboard and pen so I could communicate and she suggested we played a game in which we had to draw a film and the other one guess what it was.

So you start with the obvious ones: a shark's fin above some waves for *Jaws*, a brick road for *The Wizard of Oz*.

Then for two hours we carried on, sometimes joined by a nurse peering past my drip to see my infantile attempt to draw a bicycle passing the moon and shouting, '*E.T.*!'

My daughter drew a trilby hat next to a mushroom cloud. '*Oppenheimer*,' I wrote, though what I was actually expressing as I wrote it was 'OPPENHEIMER, YES, GOT IT.'

One of us, I can't remember which, drew a person splattered at the bottom of a cliff.

'*Midsommar*,' the other one either shouted or wrote, and we both laughed until the other patients looked across with that cocktail of curiosity and joy you feel when you see people giggling uncontrollably at something hidden from you.

Throughout this time I must have regularly spat globules into a salad bowl, and had my drip altered from water to chemicals to chemo. I must have been to the toilet while dragging my drip and felt my neck burning crisply away. But all I recall of those two hours is a beautiful period of laughter with my daughter, so I would without hesitation go through that exact experience any time it was offered with nothing altered, and I would like to thank my cancer for that.

Nine

We Should Be Friends

I sent a message to Matt Forde, who told me that on the night we'd had a drink in Edinburgh he'd decided not to mention that he was worried he might have cancer as it would spoil the night. And so both of us had been stood in the Pleasance Courtyard thinking the same thoughts.

It's so often the case that when you're worried about saying something, in fact it turns out the other person is thinking exactly the same.

Matt had cancer in the bones in his back, so he was due for an operation on the same day as mine. It would save his life, he'd been told, but he would lose bladder and bowel functions for ever. He'd also be unable to walk for a while but would relearn that with a bit of physio. I told him he'd have to learn to walk on crutches in the style of Donald Trump and Keir Starmer.

And when he was coming round from his operation he might think he's Michael Gove, doing it so convincingly the surgeons believe him.

Later we sent each other progress reports, him learning to walk and me learning to swallow. And he told me one nurse mistakenly told him they'd 'sewn my arsehole up', adding, 'I want to keep it going, even if it's only for show.' He said he feared it would become like one of these old London Underground stations that's been shut down, so there are tunnels down there but no one has seen them for many years.

Looking back at the messages we sent each other, about two-thirds of mine are positive but all of his were full of optimism and flowing with relief at his survival with not a hint of regret or lament for his bowels, bladder or (temporarily) his legs.

I wondered whether this was the reaction of a soul that hadn't yet come to terms with the reality and at some point he would crash. But he just carried on being so positive and cheerful it became almost infuriating. If I sent him a slightly frustrated message to say I'd been up all night coughing, he would reply that was a shame, but he'd had a marvellous day as he'd been learning how to sit up and had made a bit of progress.

When I told him my voice had gone, he replied that if it didn't come back he could impersonate me and ruin my credentials by making me say I'd supported the war in Iraq.

We agreed that between us we had a whole human being, and we could even go for a pint as long as he drank it and I pissed it out.

Each time he sent a message it appeared like a little beacon. There's nothing like cancer for making friends.

*

There's a wonderful saying that it takes a village to raise a child. Similarly, it takes a village to get someone through cancer.

You could argue it takes two villages, as there's the team at the hospital who diagnose you, analyse you, treat you and cure you. Then there's the network of people who are a sporadic array of close friends and acquaintances, collected throughout a lifetime from living near them, working with them and giggling somewhere together so you stay in touch for 40 years.

There are so many people who added to the gaiety of my sickness. They all combined to create the moments that not only get you through each day, but make you *want* to get through each day.

I hesitate to give anyone any advice about anything, but here's my tip if you know someone who lands in a serious medical condition.

If you're not sure what to say to someone, don't worry because anything you say is better than nothing. I can't remember the exact words of many of the messages I got; I can only remember that they came.

Every email, text or call is a reminder that you matter to someone, and that is critical in getting you past the difficult moments.

Don't worry about saying the wrong thing. All the person remembers is that you got in touch.

If you send a message that goes, 'Hello, I hope you're alright,' no one will think, *IS THAT IT? For GOD's sake, you would think that upon hearing about my condition they might pen some carefully worded prose rounded off with a sonnet, the twat.*

For example, I was especially grateful to my neighbours, because a few days before my operation, we had a discussion in which they asked if I could get my apple tree cut back so they would get more light at the bottom of their garden. I said I would sort it at some point but it was awkward at the moment because I had cancer and was having my first operation the next Monday.

On Monday evening as I sifted through the long list of

adorable messages, I found one from the neighbour that said, 'Hope the operation went well. Have you thought any more about cutting back the tree?'

*

When someone visits during your sickness, who you've always had a fairly equal relationship with, joking with each other, popping round each other's houses, taking it in turns to buy drinks or pay for tea and cake, it's hard not to feel guilty when they're making all the effort, while you sit there lazily coughing and dipping your head into a bowl of steam.

One day just before Christmas, my friends Paul and Vissy visited. As they came in, I tried to say 'Hello' but started coughing. I sat on the settee, still coughing, always feeling the cough would soon be over and I could get on with saying 'hello'. But it went on, getting stronger, until I was blasting and frothing mucus into the salad bowl. This went on for 20 minutes while they offered to help and I could only nod until eventually they wished me well and left. I've never read one of these books about the etiquette of hosting guests but I doubt whether I followed many of the rules on that day.

The next day, Christmas Eve, Vissy knocked at the door with her sister and sang a medley of Christmas carols, then without a word, she left.

It was a wonderful satire on illness and Christmas, a parody of the shows in which someone like Noel Edmonds tours a children's ward wearing a Santa hat covered in tinsel.

I'd known my dear friends Hugh and Jan since we were neighbours 40 years earlier in a road of squats. Over the following months, they came with me to scans, biopsies, endoscopies and meetings with consultants.

There were two days after I'd returned from hospital when my son had to go abroad, so Hugh stayed with me. He hadn't seen *Squid Game* so we watched the whole series, which allowed us to pretend this was all normal and we were simply enjoying a lazy couple of days watching television and cancer was nothing to do with any of it.

Fatima the French teacher came to a meeting with a consultant and my friend Julian the pianist sent me a wonderful playlist of jazz piano.

The comedian Seann Walsh asked me about the outcome of a meeting with the doctor, so I told him they'd put me in a category of 'high expectation of cure'. I started to explain the details and he said, 'Alright, no one wants to know all that bollocks, if you're going to be cured that's all we need.' Then he hung up.

Dozens of people contacted me on social media to say they'd been through radiotherapy, and it was all a bit tricky but they were fine now and wished me luck. This was especially inspiring as I thought, *Everyone who goes through this seems to come out fine in the end.*

Eventually it occurred to me I wasn't likely to get many messages saying, 'I had radiotherapy for cancer five years ago. Unfortunately it didn't work and I died four years ago, but best of luck.'

*

Two days before Christmas, as my voice waned into its state of hibernation for the winter, my agent asked if it was alright to give my number to a comic who wanted to call me. I said that was fine and a few moments later I answered the phone to Jimmy Tarbuck.

Jimmy Tarbuck was one of the classic gag tellers who became enormously famous in the early days of television when 15 million people watched either BBC or ITV every night.

He appeared on all the shows there were, like Sunday Night at the Palladium and This Is Your Life. He had his own show and in 1970 was probably better known in Britain than President Nixon or the Pope.

So when the new era of comedy began in the late 1970s, he was the personification of the enemy, a figurehead, much as an anarchist revolution would have made its chief targets President Nixon and the Pope.

Then in 1983 he appeared at an election rally alongside Margaret Thatcher. That was IT. Now he'd REALLY gone too far.

Around 1988 I was asked to appear on his show and politely declined, as that would be collaborating with the occupying army.

Twenty years later the distinctions between comic eras had become much less distinct. Most of the previous generation acknowledged the reasons they'd been usurped and a lasting truce was agreed.

Which was just as well, because I was in an Uber on the way to radiotherapy, listening to Jimmy Tarbuck tell me he'd been moved when he read about my illness and could tell I was a comic because I'd said the cancer was a nuisance, but on the other hand I'd get at least an hour of material out of it.

He'd gone to some lengths to contact me and as we wound our way through south London, I listened to this man in his eighties who I had once considered a demon acting out of sincere generosity and kindness.

If I'd read that he was ill, would I have found his number and called him? Of course not.

With my frail vocal cords I thanked him and decided this wasn't the time to debate Thatcherite monetary policy, as he drifted into a story about the advice Tommy Cooper gave him before a Royal Variety show.

I coughed for a few minutes into a salad bowl and felt everything would be alright with the world.

*

What are you supposed to do if a friend tells you they have cancer? Many people ask, 'Is there anything I can do?' But it's a difficult question to answer. Sometimes I wanted to reply by saying, 'You haven't got a cure, have you?'

I remember being on the other side of things when Jeremy and Linda were going through it. Would I follow a similar route to them? It felt I'd been so ignorant of Linda's predicament. I didn't ever ask her about the details of appointments, the different departments she was sent to, the way so many people did with me. I let her tell me as if I was a soldier instructed on a need-to-know basis.

How do you know the right amount to ask and to offer and to interfere? There were times when I appreciated people asking about the details and predictions, and other times when I found the same questions a nuisance. Cancer patients are fickle bastards.

Six years earlier, Jeremy and I went to a BBC radio Christmas party and after a few beers he told me how much weight he'd lost. 'That's good,' I said, as I knew he'd been to the gym a lot.

'But I shouldn't be losing this much,' he said, 'these trousers are so loose.'

'You look better every year,' said a writer who overheard, who then pointed at me and added, 'not like this scruffy bastard.'

He always had a complaint about his digestion or his bowel movements, his bladder or his nasal passage, and a few months later he mentioned a lump below his throat that the doctors would have to take out at some point and examine. But he didn't want to do it just yet as he was on tour and had a run of radio shows coming up, so he delayed procedures that might have told us about his condition sooner.

Would it have made a difference if I'd said to him after the Christmas party, 'WHAT DO YOU MEAN, YOU'RE LOSING LOADS OF WEIGHT? GET YOURSELF TO THE DOCTOR NOW, YOU TWAT.'

Philosophers and therapists may say there's no point in wondering; you can only damage yourself by regretting what can't be changed.

But it's a question that won't ever fully go away.

You could always approach a cancerous friend in the manner of Seann Walsh, who saw me just after the diagnosis and gave me a packet of Strepsils, saying, 'That should sort it,' while laughing uncontrollably.

One of the most useful things you can do if you have a friend with cancer is to have had cancer yourself.

My friend Pat went further than this, because as well as having had throat cancer four years earlier, he was born with no legs and one arm, so when I spoke to him I had no way of feeling sorry for myself.

Pat was the first person I knew who had cancer and came through it. When he told me about his diagnosis, my first thought was the traditional one of 'Oh. So how long will it be before you die then?'

He had a course of radiotherapy, during which time he felt awful for three of the six weeks it lasted, but he told me he was never so exhausted that he missed a Spurs home game.

In the early weeks of my adventure I asked him about the details of his treatment and he told me about the uncertainty of the weeks before the diagnosis, the nervousness of the meetings, the mask, the whirring, clunking machine, the serenity of the Macmillan Cancer Centre and how it had taken him an hour to eat a Weetabix.

Maybe the best thing he did of all was to be there. I don't mean in the sense that 'he was there for me, staying strong'. I mean he was there, literally there, watching sport, listening to music and infuriated by the government, discussing the details of his radiotherapy as a temporary ordeal that was endured long ago, the way you might remember a few months when the heating didn't work.

The comic Rhod Gilbert had been through a far greater bashing, in which the cancer had arrived in four separate places. He told me the consultant said to him, 'This will be a significant bump in your journey, but we hope it won't be your last,' which I suppose is another way of saying 'touch wood'.

Rhod had patiently relayed the likely course I would enjoy: the coughing, the vomiting, the mucus, exhaustion, tears, despair, fractious endless nights, unforeseen dramatic complications and eventual triumphant cure.

He talked about booking an Airbnb next to the hospital towards the end of his treatment, as he didn't have the energy to get there from home.

I was immensely grateful for the parameters suggested by these contrasting experiences; mine ended up being somewhere in the middle.

There's also the camaraderie that came from others. During the week when my biopsy had gone missing, as we were warming up for a game of football, my friend Daniel asked if I was in some ways reassured by how incompetent the system seemed to be.

I suppose he meant that if the system made mistakes, it was possible they'd got everything wrong and there was nothing wrong with me at all.

But another friend heard this and exclaimed, 'Oh, of course, when you've got a life-threatening illness, what you want above all else is that the people in charge of it are all utterly incompetent, the more useless the better.

Hopefully they get your name wrong and treat you for the wrong condition.'

And as I stood there laughing, Daniel yelled, 'Right, I hope you've got a really bad cancer and that he catches it off you.'

It was a model of what to say to someone fearing they had cancer, and it should be in an NHS handbook

The people I'd known for years had been friends in that we'd met up for a laugh over thousands of coffees or pints of beer. We'd seen bands and sporting events together, done shows and podcasts and TV or radio shows together, seen each other in bars and at parties and during the festival in Edinburgh, been to each other's weddings and gone for curries during each other's divorces. Now they were accompanying me to meetings with surgeons and consultants in which my short-term fate was presented in a tiny office.

They would come to see me, in the hospital or in my living room, to ask how I was and laugh when I told them, with no excuse for being in my presence such as a concert or a beer or a curry or a chat about a script. This takes a bit of getting used to.

They were just there to see me. Because they wanted to improve my day. I felt a bit guilty, like I should at least have booked a band to play in the kitchen.

For 35 years I'd written scripts with Pete. Then we made a podcast together.

But now he was popping round to watch me spluttering into a bowl. Then he came to collect me from the hospital when I was sent home after they'd fitted my nose tube.

My instinct was to pretend as far as possible that everything was normal. I wanted to say, 'Once we get home and I've fed myself through a syringe into my nose, and had a sleep to recover from a week in hospital and I'm no longer so exhausted I have to stop for a breath on the way to the toilet, we can get on with working on this script.'

It's difficult to accept that your friends are there just to care for you. It feels so imbalanced.

It seems there's a seamless shift from the everyday relationships you have with the network of people around you. Normally they consist of natural jokey conversation and frivolous jollity, but suddenly this transforms into a commitment to urgent action.

It's as if the circle of people around us are an army in a peaceful state, often unseen for long periods, usually strolling calmly, occasionally getting a bit raucous, but when there's a crisis, suddenly mobilising all their battalions and sweeping into action.*

*

During the most vicious week of assaults on the body, the Stalingrad of my time with cancer, a variety of cards and notes were delivered, including a parcel that I was only vaguely aware of. Penetrating the obstinate cardboard seemed like one more unnecessary task to be added to the schedule. I have no idea how long it was before I attended

* I'm aware that analogy works only for kindly armies that exist solely in the imagination, not the real ones that invade Iraq or Ukraine.

to it, maybe a whole day. I probably put it on my lap several times but was distracted by the usual kaleidoscope of bodily breakdowns.

Eventually I discovered a *Viz* annual. I poked inside for a card, a letter, some indication of the sender, but there was none. It was the perfect gift for the time. If I was to be able to read anything it would be an episode of the Drunken Bakers or the Fat Slags, with plots that could be absorbed in four quick bursts between coughing fits, with delicate shifts of the eyes as I couldn't move my crispy neck, in a way that might not be possible with a Zola novel.

It was a perfect anonymous cancer treatment gift, the measured piece of culture I needed, as I laughed silently at the Top Tips and Mrs Brady Old Lady and hoped that whoever sent it would be aware of my gratitude.

*

On the first day of my radiotherapy I sat in the chair waiting to be called in, acknowledging my co-cancerees. There were a few of us starting at the same time, so we would nod to each other over the next six weeks as we passed in the corridor. There was a sturdy-looking Polish man who noticed my scarf. 'Football,' he said, pointing at it.

'Yes, Crystal Palace,' I said.

'Arsenal,' he replied, tapping himself on the chest.

Throughout the following weeks we communicated by saying 'Crystal Palace' or 'Arsenal', then smiling or pulling a face, depending on the result of the previous day's game. I have no idea how he is.

There was a man who said nothing at all, not even to his wife who came in with him every day, and as the treatment wore on he said even less than the nothing he'd started with.

There was a boy of about 13 who had no hair, which I guessed was due to chemotherapy, but I didn't get a chance to talk to him. And a Hasidic Jewish man whose son came every day, who would stand in the corridor reading out loud what I presume were texts from the Torah that were printed on a sheet of paper, as the whirring and beeping flowed from the radiotherapy room. I told him I loved his black wide-brimmed hat, but avoided the more difficult subjects such as whether it's considered insulting to wear a hat like that if you're not a Hasidic Jew, and what sort of cancer he had.

And there was a man called Jules who told me he was a fan of my radio show. Jules and I shared a trait of describing most experiences through the medium of sport, so after the first day of treatment I suggested this first few days was all about seeing off the opening bowlers, and he described the results of his operation as an ugly 2–1 win. We pledged to get through the six weeks of radiotherapy without ever taking the lift back up to the ground floor, but always walking up the four flights of steps, even if it took 15 minutes. Each day we'd describe the previous day's climb as 'set off at a good pace but only the first stage of the Tour de France'. By the third week it was 'two sets and a break down with a heavily bandaged ankle, but determined to finish the match'.

I asked Jules if he found the first day of wearing the mask a bit claustrophobic and he replied that he had a bit of experience of confined spaces, as he'd been a tank commander in the army and there's not as much space as you'd think in a tank. He was now a general in the army, with a CBE, and I didn't know many of them.

He said it had helped to read the Stoics. 'What, like Marcus Aurelius?' I suggested. 'Yes, that's the sort of thing,' he said. 'You can dip in and out of it.'

And that's true, because the writings offer a calm assertion of the benefits of accepting what you can't control, which is a valuable sentiment during cancer treatment, whatever other issues you may have with someone who was a Roman emperor.

It wasn't where I thought our conversation would go, as he described some of the treatment he'd already undergone. A long operation had taken a slice of his quadriceps to rebuild his face and neck after removing tumours.

It had taken a while to recover from this and now he was ready to embark on the next stage of treatment, along with the rest of us novice radiotherapees, but more than any of us he was 'looking to be positive', like a footballer refusing to despair in an interview after a 4–0 defeat.

Jules is a competitive rower and, in a display of extreme positivity, on the day before his radiotherapy began he bought a new racing boat (a single scull, which sounds ambitious if you had no tumours at all).

'Whatever happens, I want to leave something positive for my kids out of it,' he told me, which seemed remarkably stoic.

During the third week of the treatment, as everything from the neck upwards ground to a halt, we checked each other's progress or decline and measured it against our own. During week four when he confessed he'd suddenly felt his body was breaking down, I was relieved because it made me feel we were both in step. Then I felt horrible that my thought process, in effect, was, *That's marvellous! Hopefully he can barely walk!* Sometimes we recommended creams, medicines or steaming techniques that were working for us and discussed which exercises were still manageable.

Jules and I shared an idea of holding a Christmas party in the summer when all this would be over, and as the symptoms of treatment faded we discussed how the mucus and the burning was replaced by anxiety about the post-treatment scan.

I told him I was going to Stoke for my *In Town* series, a city that seemed to have been battered more than almost any other by neglect and unemployment. And he replied that he'd been there a few times, as it was one of the best places to sign up recruits to the army. He marched around the town with his regiment, exercising its freedom of the city.

We were from such different worlds. But now we shared the same one: outside booth D of the radiotherapy unit at UCH.

We'll stay in touch for the rest of our lives.

Ten

Just Be

Moaning has a hierarchy and if you don't follow it you very quickly become annoying. It probably isn't fair but it's unavoidable.

A couple of years before my diagnosis I was talking to my friend, the comic and ridiculously knowledgeable expert on music, Mark Lamarr. He'd been reading about the Stoics, he said: 'And they argue that nobody can annoy you. The source of your annoyance is always you, because you have chosen to be annoyed by them.' Then he added, 'I don't think I've ever read anything as annoying as that.'

By the third week, as the mucus started to flow and cannulas and endoscopies bounced in and out of me, I had become proficient at attaining a calm state of acceptance, submitting to whatever procedure was necessary, no longer cringing or tightening as I once would have done; I had now meekly surrendered like one of the locusts I used to watch in a cage, apparently without concern as it sat on the back of my daughter's pet lizard, waiting to be eaten.

The sting, the poke, the jolt would happen in a moment, then it would be over and the only influence I had on it was to decide whether to make it worse by resisting and making it last twice as long, or to make moaning noises and ask why this was happening to me, as if it was a personal message from God, maybe as revenge for writing those sketches in my TV show about Charles Darwin.

I'd think about the man with the arsenic drip and everyone else I kept running into who were going through it too and I did as almost all patients learn to do, and accepted that at a certain level we experience the pain we choose to experience. This doesn't mean the pain isn't real – the nerves are being prodded and the brain does receive the messages that this fucking hurts – but you can reach a state you might not have thought you were capable of, in which you regard this as necessary, it will pass and therefore it strangely doesn't hurt as much. Marcus Aurelius and the Stoics fetishised it more than I did, but one of the advantages of having had cancer is that I have a fuller understanding of what they were on about than I did before.

So I took Jules's advice and read Marcus's *Meditations*, which he wrote partly while he was emperor, which suggests the job of Roman emperor wasn't quite as time-consuming as you might think. He insisted regularly in his book that 'we must accept without resentment whatever may befall'.

'Without resentment'! That's not easy, because truly terrible things can befall that it would take an extraordinary soul not to resent.

But he pursues this repeatedly. 'Put from you the belief that "I have been wronged" and with it will go the feeling. Reject your sense of injury, and the injury itself disappears.'

Again, this might be taking it a bit further than I'd be prepared to go. I don't think I'd have trusted a consultant who told me if I rejected the sense of the cancer, it would disappear (although it would have been no less scientific than the plan of action that began 'touch wood').

But the sense of injustice about the cancer can be made to disappear.

The Stoics didn't just advocate this philosophy of living as a series of pithy statements to put on Instagram or embroider onto a piece of cloth so it could be framed and hung on an office wall.

They believed the soul lives on after death, in the upper regions of the air, until a final conflagration (a bit like the Day of Judgement).

To follow the 'advice' of the Stoics without acknowledging their religious origins would make a nonsense of everything they say. But to reject their attitude because it springs from a religious source would be nonsensical as well. It would be like dismissing the speeches of Martin Luther King because he believed racism was fundamentally an affront to God as he'd made all men equal.

And they certainly hit upon a way of thinking that inhabited my mind during my cancer period, that resentment and bitterness at illness is not only futile but counterproductive.

It fascinated me that most patients I encountered seemed to arrive close to this point, possibly without reading Marcus Aurelius. The bald Cockney man in the chemo room, the over-cheerful soul in the hospital, the man in the bed opposite, Jules, the man whose only English was football teams: they all exuded a robust cocktail of resignation and determination.

'When anything tempts you to feel bitter,' said Marcus, 'think not "this is a misfortune", but "to bear this worthily is good fortune".'

If I were writing that I might try to sound a little less pompous, but as this was written in Latin 1,900 years ago we should probably accept the translation might not be exact.

But there's no doubt that bitterness is not your friend.

The stoicism I saw in the people I met was not the modern attitude of ignoring emotions and pledging to 'carry on regardless', like a First World War general advising a 17-year-old who's just seen 20 of his mates splattered in the mud to 'try not to dwell on it'; it was an acceptance that fate is not out to get you and if we try to deal with each situation there's so much to be gained from even the most difficult of days.

What I didn't appreciate until around nine months after my treatment ended was how I was still trying to think like that.

For example, one section of the *Meditations* begins, 'Do not waste what remains of your life by speculating about neighbours, what so-and-so is doing, what he is saying or thinking ... That men of a certain type should behave as they do is inevitable. To wish it otherwise is to wish the fig-tree did not yield its juice.'

So this is very positive, but then to emphasise his point he adds, 'In any case remember that in a very little while both of you will be dead.'

Which spoils the optimistic nature of the sentiment a bit.

But this is a recurring theme, that allowing our thoughts, emotions and efforts to be dominated by the actions of others that we can't control is particularly damaging because soon, cancer or no cancer, WE'LL ALL BE DEAD.

Marcus Aurelius had worked out through philosophy what I had to learn from having cancer. If I'd translated that sentence it would say, 'Time is finite so don't waste it getting in a flap about a row with the neighbour over a tree.'

He repeats this sentiment often, saying, 'Understand your time has a limit to it, use it then, or it will be gone and never in your power again.'

I love the phrase 'never in your power again'. You have a superpower, which is to be able to use time. And one day that superpower will be gone.

Unlike most modern self-help books, this all seems supremely rooted in the material world. It could apply to a trade union campaign for improved nurses' pay as much as a plea to write an epic poem or repair your relationship with your father.

Occasionally you hear someone comment that 'it isn't fair' that a particular person has cancer. It's a kind sentiment but makes no sense for me. Fairly early on in life it should become clear there's no sense of fairness in illness or human circumstances.

You'd have to be very naive to believe there's a link between merit and severe illness.

There aren't many circumstances in which someone can say, 'You know Eric who runs the printer's on the corner? He's got cancer. At least that's fair because he's a cunt.'

I'd seen two of my closest friends dissolve like this. Did that make me unlucky? Or did it make me lucky because I was still fit and healthy? I was 63 years old when I was diagnosed with cancer, so in a global sense I was already past the average life expectancy. If you assess luck by taking into account everyone in history going back to the Stone Age, I was among the luckiest people ever.

For me the concept of fairness is relevant once there's a decision made by someone. It isn't fair that you should have to pay a parking fine if your tyre is six inches over the little line. And it isn't fair that millions of people suffer from illness because they live in an area of the world in which there's a shortage of food, water and basic healthcare. Because it should be relatively simple to provide that, but the world's food, water and basic healthcare is run by people who don't prioritise getting it to people who can't pay for it.

But the allocation of cancer is mostly a random act of nature. You can improve your odds through exercise or worsen them by smoking or rolling around in nuclear waste, but the main factor that determines whether you get cancer and how damaging it is will be luck.

Even if you believe that illness is governed by an interventionist god, you must have noticed that the kindest souls tend not to be rewarded with longer, healthier lives than the horrible bastards.

Disputing the fairness of who gets cancer may even be counterproductive. I can't imagine how much extra stress you put on yourself, if every time you're asked by a nurse to lie back so she can prod you, your mind is occupied by thoughts of how unfair it all is that you're here at all.

If you're detained as a political prisoner you probably need a different set of priorities. I suppose you endeavour to stay calm but also retain a burning sense of injustice against Putin or the Chinese government or whoever put you there. But if you have cancer there's no advantage in seething about your cells for mutating, the vicious organisms, and pledging that one day you'll defeat them and their rotten system.

I have always found it dispiriting when I hear other comics complaining that 'it's not fair how THAT person has got on *Live at the Apollo* and not me' or lament that their career has stagnated because some other comic does a similar act to them. But now I want to scream at them, 'STOP IT! Do what YOU think is worth doing in whatever forum is available to do it, even if it's the local church hall, and STOP COMPLAINING.'

And having read the *Meditations* I would add, 'Because in a very little while you will be dead.'

To which I suppose I couldn't blame them if they said, 'I don't think I've ever heard anything as annoying as that.'

You can't complain too much about the debilitating effects of an itchy backside to someone who's in a wheelchair.

Or splutter through a panic attack that Sainsbury's delivered the wrong groceries and Colin's mum is coming round tomorrow and you've got no aubergines and so you broke down and cried, if you're talking to a refugee who's just arrived from Belgium on an inflatable lilo.

Once you've got cancer, you're in a different place in the moaning ladder.

During my last trips out to a pub or cafe before the treatment, if I heard someone at another table spluttering something like, 'We've had the builders in for the last three weeks and it's been UNBEARABLE, we have to squeeze past some bags of plaster to get to the downstairs bathroom, it's ABSOLUTE HELL,' I'd be tempted to play my cancer card, and lean across to bark, 'I'll show you something to moan about, you miserable twat.'

I've always been slightly infuriated by the lack of perspective at the heart of most minor domestic turmoil.

But now, if I heard a squeal of 'We've had SUCH problems with our neighbours, their bush has grown over a foot since we moved in and it casts a shadow over our hydrangeas so they're not getting enough sunlight but they refuse to cut it down and I've paid for a solicitor to write to them and now they ignore me in the street,' I'd feel entitled to yell, 'Oh FUCK OFF. I hope their bush grows another foot tonight and spurts shaving foam all over your fucking flowers and they all shrivel up so you dig them up and discover your garden's built on the burial ground of a Native American tribe and now you've disturbed their spirits so you're cursed so you can't even sell the house and you try to claim on the insurance but it turns out there's a clause that any damage caused by the people of the Iroquois renders your policy null and void.' I never did say anything like that, or mention that I had cancer to any strangers. And with my newfound stoicism, other people's complaints about everyday life didn't annoy me as much as I expected, as I couldn't expect that no one in the world would ever again be annoyed by anything less dramatic than cancer. I just wanted to use my opportunity while it was there.

But I can't think of a single moment when I was able to employ my cancer status to any effect. I couldn't settle an argument with it, or move up a space in any queue, or even embarrass someone who had shoved their way past me in some way. Maybe there have been patients who have waited to be seated at a restaurant and said softly to the waiter, 'Could we jump ahead of this couple, please? I've got cancer.' Or explained to a dealer in a car showroom, 'I've got cancer, so can you drop the price another £300?'

The only times I got to mention my health to someone who didn't ask was when I really needed it for an excuse. During some of the Uber journeys to my radiotherapy sessions, I would sit on the back seat and pour my frothy spit into my salad bowl, feeling the poor driver's tension as he wondered how long it would take to scrub his seat if I missed the bowl, and whether my spit was full of an unknown alien acid and would burn through his whole car and make a pothole in the road. 'Sorry,' I whispered, 'it's to do with cancer.'

Each time the driver nodded sympathetically, while watching me closely in the mirror to check I was hitting the middle of the bowl.

Eleven

Can't Get Out of Bed

I was still in theory in a state that might be called 'dating'. I hadn't seen the person I was 'dating' for a few weeks, especially over Christmas, as she had her family round and a family Christmas is too easily spoilt by the sounds of a man coughing and vomiting in the attic. As I reached the advanced burning steaming phase of my treatment, that was now accompanied by my voice having disappeared, she called me on FaceTime to ask why I hadn't replied to a text message she'd sent that morning.

So I mimed that I'd been syringing some bottles, trying not to mime in a way that looked sarcastic. Then followed a conversation that was a little one-sided, though I did spit into the salad bowl a couple of times. She asked me to do that a bit to the left so I was out of shot and she told me she felt the situation had been a little one-sided lately.

I texted to say that was probably a fair assessment and she asked me more questions so I looked back blankly. There are many times when I've not been sure what to say to someone, but this was the first time I was sure what I needed to say to someone, which was 'I can't answer you because I literally can't speak', but couldn't say it as I literally couldn't speak.

I texted 'I'm sorry, I can't speak' and then she hung up and that was pretty much the last contact we had.

The worst part was I couldn't really blame her.

Occasionally I see a discussion on a TV show in which people compete to recount stories of dates that have gone horribly wrong. But I reckon with my one, I'd have a very good chance of getting to at least the semi-final.

*

I was warned many times by all the doctors, consultants and nurses that after the treatment is finished, I should expect the impact to get worse for two more weeks. So I was prepared for 'things' to get 'worse', but this all seemed a bit vague. In what way would they be worse?

Would the 'things' already happening get stronger, and the mucus start pouring out of my ears and backside too?

Or would there be new 'things', so I could only walk like a chicken, or I'd start hovering over the bed and vomiting green sticky paste and develop the ability to make priests fly backwards out of the window?

Friends would congratulate me on the approaching end of the treatment. 'Nearly over, you're almost finished,' they'd say, and in my drowsy stupor I would try and show I appreciated their kind thoughts and not make it look like I was thinking, *I'm nowhere near finished, it gets worse, your cheery optimism is entirely misplaced.*

One morning around 7.30 I stood at the top of the stairs, aiming to perform my daily tasks, then get to the hospital for the treatment.

After each step I felt compelled to have a rest so I told myself to keep forging ahead, in a 'search for the hero inside yourself' way, reaching for untapped residues of grit and determination to overcome all obstacles, shrugging off pain like a cyclist on the steepest of Alps in the Tour de France.

That allowed me to reach the second step, where I clung to the banister for two minutes.

At the bottom of the steps I could turn on the television, have another rest and wait for enough energy to arrive so I could start syringing. But an episode of *Friends* appeared and I watched it all, justifying it as I needed the rest. As soon as it ended, I would feed myself and get up to go to the hospital.

Then another episode came on so I amended my plan to the end of that one, and then I gazed at three more. Slowly I boiled a kettle, rested, had to boil it again, put my head in the steam, then the hospital called to ask where I was.

Now it felt exactly like my job in a London Transport office in 1982, when every morning I trod the line between dreading my arrival there as I hated every moment, and dreading not getting there because I'd get a call from the fearful Mrs Bartlett who would demand to know where I was.

'I'm sorry,' I mouthed, but the woman from radiotherapy reception couldn't hear that.

She soothingly urged me to get there before they closed for the evening, with a compassion I couldn't recall from Mrs Bartlett. She was so sympathetic and patient as I texted my plight that I felt a tear forming, because nothing seems to move the human spirit as much as a stranger's kindness in a moment that you'd written off as hopeless.

I arrived about four hours late for my appointment and if they hadn't shown me gently into a room to give me extra medication, I'd have spluttered, 'I'm really sorry but as I was about to leave the house I felt a terrible stomach ache so I went to the doctor and I couldn't phone in sick because I had cramp in my fingers and then the train went the wrong way and I promise I'll be on time tomorrow, Mrs Bartlett,' except I'd have moved my lips and no sound would have come out.

*

Jeremy and I met up a few times during his treatment and then he disappeared for two weeks, which was very out of character. Like the owner of an old frail cat that knows something's wrong when it goes missing, I sensed some darkness. Eventually he answered when I called, chatted about the absurdity of Boris Johnson for a while and then said, 'Oh, the cancer situation isn't good,' just like Linda and as if he was lamenting that the exhaust on his car had broken down.

The cancer was in his bones, and it was somewhere else that I didn't really grasp, just that it was somewhere and they could try and shrink it and operate on it but it would probably be fatal within two years.

The simplicity of the way he said this added to the thud of the effect. There was no waffle, nothing an editor needed to cut, it was basic and thorough and final.

I had to tell other comics and his agent, and some would resist the reality. I heard several sentences that began 'maybe there's a trial ...' or 'they don't always know with these things ...' And maybe that's always possible, but there was something bleakly definite about Jeremy's words, as certain as the look on the person who's packed their bags and are really leaving and there's no point in arguing.

Over the next few months I went with him to see dentists and oncologists and sat round his house while he had chemotherapy at home, which seemed quite a luxury.

I spoke to him about making a podcast as there were so many stories, memories and anecdotes that I feared would be lost. But the cancer ripped through him too fast and by the start of December it had reached his brain.

The day after he discovered this, I went to his home where I mentioned our mate Seann, who was in the newspapers for a scandal about kissing his dancer on *Strictly Come Dancing*. I told Jeremy that the national furore had affected Seann and he said, 'Mark, there are problems, and then there are problems.'

Over the next few weeks I watched Jeremy's final demise, saw him pool all his resolve to hold a rapid pop-up wedding with his wife, and give his daughter away at her own instantly organised marriage.

I sat with him through hospital appointments in which he was told there were only weeks left and saw him nod, as if he was listening to a plumber explaining he needed new radiators.

We continued to discuss Brexit and comedy and we spent a while trying to stop his Christmas tree from wobbling and in those moments you wonder if you should be doing something more profound. But maybe carrying on as close to normal for as long as possible is what we all want to do. If you discovered you had a week to live, you probably wouldn't want someone to let off fireworks every time you spoke, or stand beside you reading sonnets.

What can you do when someone you love is dying? You

carry on as normal apart from when you can't, because they have to be carried down the stairs or tipped into a car from a wheelchair.

I sat in the hospice with his wife, daughter and another friend as he eased through his last hours, and he left us on an icy January night. Was this the saddest moment, or was that the moment when he told me this day was imminent?

A couple of hours after he died, as we sat with his body, a woman of about 30 who worked there came in. She looked at the full glass next to his bed and said, 'Oh, he hasn't drunk his water.'

'No,' I said, 'he does seem to have left it.'

'Do you think he'll want it later?' she asked.

'I think the odds are against it,' I said, 'but you never know.'

'I'll leave it there just in case,' she said.

And when she left the room we all laughed, as it would have been very rude not to.

Later that morning I sat in my local cafe with my laptop, as I so often did, but this time to write an obituary.

While I was there the obituary writer from *The Times* called and said he'd like to 'ask some questions about Mr Hardy'.

'Of course,' I said.

'Firstly,' he said, 'was Jeremy political in any way?'

I was so flummoxed, with this strange question on top of the morning's events, that I said, 'Yes, well, yes.'

'Good,' he said, like a doctor examining tonsils. 'Next, was he a keen sportsman?'

'Not really,' I said.

As soon as I put the phone down I was furious with myself for not saying, 'He was Chairman of the East Surrey Conservative Association and played rugby league to a semi-professional standard.'

Because if that had gone in *The Times* to be seen for ever, it would have been the nearest Jeremy would get to drawing a cock and balls all over one of its inside pages.

*

Two days after my last radiotherapy I was aware I felt worse. I was more tired than I'd been for months, and after a shower and cleaning my teeth I felt dizzy and had to sit down to get my breath back.

Ulcers popped up in assorted regions of my mouth, which stung and throbbed and sometimes went to sleep so I'd forget they were there or even imagine they'd disappeared, then re-emerged, invigorated by their rest, and zinged across my tongue and throat with piercing, pulsating jolts of venom.

And the mucus came from a deeper place, a new level rooted in the centre of my being; it came out in globular lumps between the size of a marble and a meatball. These would emerge in one plop, as if fired by a paintball gun, pure and untroubled by anything in its way. They would ping out in one motion and land perfectly in the sink or toilet bowl, and I imagined a team of judges holding up cards to show a very creditable 5.8 for a clinical dive and very straight entry.

This was the week when there was barely any moment

without discomfort, just a change in which discomfort was the most discomfortable, so I would concentrate on a different area.

Coughing always trumped the others. When the cough was in control, there was no way of pausing it, it just demanded its own path, to rattle everything around the throat and the lungs, so I would shut my eyes and wait for it to pass – which eventually it must.

Then I could get back to the job of noticing the ulcers or the throat or the neck, which was crackling like a forest fire you see on the news in Australia.

Each time I saw the doctor or nurse through the period of radiotherapy, they would ask me to raise my chin so they could closely observe my neck. Studying each part in turn, they would look slightly surprised and say, 'Hmm, no real colouring yet, do you feel any burning? Hmm, not at all? Well, good, that's good.' I would take this as worthy of credit on my part. I must have been thinking, *I'm not like these normal weedy cancer patients, whose neck becomes hot and coloured because it's being irradiated on a daily basis, because my neck's clever.*

Then at the start of the sixth and final week of treatment my skin suddenly turned a satisfying blend of purple and brown, quickly enhanced with broken sore patches, and the doctors seemed almost relieved, as if they'd been opening the oven every ten minutes hoping to see an apple crumble starting to turn crisp and brown and at last it was doing what was expected.

I was given two types of cream and told to spread them across the burned region several times a day; each time I did this I was aware of the bumpy, craggy outline of my new neck, a scaled map of the Andes engraved through it, so that every time I turned in any direction I could feel it stretching and tearing and winning the temporary battle to be the discomfort that drew my attention for that moment.

Maybe the lowest point was about one week after the end of the treatment, when a sudden swirling in the stomach propelled me in two or three seconds from the settee to the kitchen sink, where I was sick through my nose and my throat and it came out in such quantities and from so many directions I assumed I must have another orifice it was splurging from, which in my haziness I'd forgotten about.

Everything felt so out of control, liquid bubbling into my mouth and flowing down the nostrils, not cleanly but murky and stuttering like the footage you see of a river bursting its banks and sweeping up branches and debris and bikes and cars, and I had no idea what was hurtling where but knew I had to get through this and in one hour I would probably feel better than this and in a week I would probably feel much better than this and my son stood next to me, occasionally asking, 'Is there anything I can do, Dad?' and I wished there was something I could have given him to do as that would have made him feel better and me feel better, but all he could do was be there, which was a huge amount by itself.

But you don't want your son seeing you dribble and involuntarily shudder and emit mucus-y nutrition-drink-based vomit across the sink where you rinse your apples and your rice.

When you're drunk or have food poisoning you can convince yourself there's a healthy side to being sick: your body is ingeniously discarding the source of its troubles. But cancer-treatment sick has no redeeming qualities; it truly is the king of all the types of sick, that other causes of sick can only look up to in wonder.

*

Luckily the World Darts Championship takes place over Christmas, the perfect sport to be watched by someone in their fifth week of radio/chemotherapy.

Jules was still eating but described the trial of eating a boiled egg as being like 'a spinner that knows they're bowling 40 overs in the heat on a wicket giving them nothing'.

By now we were creeping up the stairs from the radiotherapy lab one at a time, stopping for a rest after three steps and trying to look as if we were just admiring the view. The thought of confessing to Jules that I'd taken the lift was too traumatic to abandon this assault on the remaining steps.

One day as we waited together to see our medical teams, we had a lengthy discussion about which England cricket captains would make the best generals in the army. Botham would have been useless, we agreed, but Stokes would do the job wonderfully.

And reduced as we were to these physical states, we were able not just to watch the darts but to feel excited about it, to sense that it mattered, especially as it was the tournament in which the teenage kebab-fan Luke Littler stormed the darting world to get to the final. And so the general and I exchanged messages furiously as we made our observations on this great event.

Then the next day we'd set off up the stairs again, as if we still needed 230 while our opponent was down to a double – but you keep going, if only to get into a rhythm that can propel you to winning the next set.

Twelve

I Can See for Miles

When I bought my house, the feature that swung me was the view from the main bedroom.

Other, more pragmatic people study cupboard space and analyse whether the garden faces north or east, but I went upstairs and stared for 20 minutes through the window.

I'd already lived around the area for 25 years but this view confused me. 'Where's that airport I can see?' I asked. After 25 years you should have noticed if the local amenities include an airport.

'That's Heathrow,' said the man trying to sell the house.

He must have got that wrong; Heathrow was 20 miles away, a 90-minute drive if the traffic's bad. But across the expanse of west London, there it was. I was as amazed as if I'd asked what the pointed building was and he'd said, 'That's a pyramid.' And there was Wimbledon. And Twickenham.

My son ran up and down the stairs and my daughter, who was seven, mentioned there was plenty of cupboard space, and I knew that if I lived here, I would spend many thousands of hours gazing at that view and working out where that round tower was in the distance.

Sixteen years later, during the days and nights of erupting mucus, a flaming neck, voicelessness and vomit, I spent many hours in the toilet of that house.

In these moments I found the return to normality so distant it wasn't much comfort at all. It was too many steps away. The strategy for me was to get through today, and get closer to the end of this process. And sometimes just to get through this particular symphony of spluttering to a time when I might be able to breathe all the way in and out without an eruption.

When you're battling to just be, when every moment requires concentration – to be able to breathe, to compel your mind to bear discomfort, to make a decision about whether to leave the toilet, to turn round, to try and swallow, to reach for an inhaler – there is no space for considering anything you've read or seen or think about why and how this has all happened. You might as well expect a mouse that's cornered by a cat to use that moment to wonder how his predicament was all a result of evolution.

This must be why people who are the most downtrodden are rarely the first to create the movements that resist their plight. It's rarely the homeless or the starving who initiate the great revolts in history, although they may become energised by the sense of hope they offer. Because if you're sheltering under a bridge there isn't the space in your head to consider the long-term strategic solution to your predicament. You can only hope to find a space that protects you against the wind and get through the night. I've never been homeless, but I have been awake for 20 consecutive nights staring at the same patch of toilet bowl in a sleep-deprived haze. And I know those aren't the moments to start a discussion with someone about the paper they've written on long-term strategies for reducing mucus output during radiotherapy.

For me, the optimistic outlook was to remind myself that there will be a period of calm. It might be in 20 minutes or I may have to wait three hours, but it will come, and then I will enjoy the luxury of being alive while not having to concentrate on the functions of staying alive. I will be able to breathe in and out without thinking.

I would repeat the journey from toilet to bed and back again, again and again as if I was doing hundreds of takes of a scene in a film with a notoriously obsessive director. Eventually I would lie on the bed and after a minute or two I would find myself thinking about the film I'd seen earlier, or whether Crystal Palace would be relegated, and I'd realise my ability to think about something that wasn't immediate was back.

It always happened that way round. I started contemplating, then realised that's what I was doing. At no time did I think, *Aah, the breathing is getting better, I can start thinking again.*

During these moments of respite, that sometimes might last 30 seconds or could go on for two hours, there was a glorious peace. And the joy of those moments wasn't just an absence of discomfort. I felt wonderful. It actually felt marvellous to lie there at 3.28am breathing normally for an unspecified time, and experiencing the calm.

Through the crack in the curtains I could see the lights I'd studied, from Twickenham to Morden, and the reflections of Wimbledon and Brentford. And I was aware, because this could all be interrupted at any second, of how utterly beautiful it was.

Thirteen

The King's New Clothes

The doctors predicted I would start to feel less sick around two weeks after the radiotherapy ended. Then at around six weeks after, I would reach a 'new normal'.

This would be an exciting new world, one in which things improved. Once I was in this state, I would reasonably be able to expect that in three days' time I would feel slightly more alert and healthy. Maybe I would be spitting into a salad bowl every four minutes instead of every two minutes.

My voice might still be a rasping, grinding vinyl record being played backwards to summon the Devil, but it was more intelligible than it had been a week earlier.

This was as far ahead as it was healthy to ponder. Sometimes a friend would say, 'Just think, in no time at all we'll be going out for a curry as normal.' But that didn't feel positive. It was too utopian, no more real than if Del Boy told me that this time next year we'd be millionaires.

But if someone suggested that in a couple of weeks, I would only have to spend an hour of each day with my head under a towel nudging a bowl of boiling water with my nose, instead of an hour and a half, this presented itself as a wonderful future that I pledged to strive for.

When your body isn't functioning as it did before, you're confronted by the way all conditions are relative. If you can only sleep for three hours at a time without coughing, that feels magical after two weeks of only sleeping for two hours without coughing.

I was given a series of swallowing exercises that took around ten minutes, that the dieticians asked me to perform five times each day. One of them involved sticking your tongue out, then gently biting on it and swallowing, five times in a row. These were getting easier each day; life was improving.

Then on the ninth day after the treatment ended, I felt a strange sensation as I came down the stairs. There were bits of me that felt like they could move freely. A few breaths went all the way in, with nothing trying to prevent them. It felt like I was driving along a motorway, expecting that every time I got into third gear I'd run over one of those spiky contraptions the police throw over a road to stop getaway cars.

But instead, for the first time in two months, I just kept going. The breath flowed in and went out, and I could even walk from one room to another without pause.

Then the dieticians suggested I try sipping water. At first this seemed outlandish. I'd done well to get as far as I had, and now they were giving me superhuman tasks like that. Did they think I was one of the X-Men?

But after a week I was managing four tiny droplets, one minute apart, although the fourth one always came coughing back up. Until one morning I got as far as a fifth droplet, then a sixth. The sensation was how I imagine a professional swimmer feels if, after a month of intense training, they finally knock one tenth of a second off their time for the 200 metres butterfly.

I wanted to call everyone I knew and tell them I'd managed a sixth drop of water.

Even more significantly, I could conduct certain human activities without feeling wretched. I could have a shower that lasted two minutes without having to lean across to the sink to spit halfway through. I could tie my shoelaces without having to stop to catch my breath.

And I could speak. I called my friend Seann, who said he was amazed to hear my voice after several weeks of silence, but was also disappointed, because he'd hoped it would come back as a comedy Chinese voice from the 1970s, so the word would go round that I'd been cured of cancer but I'd been cancelled.

Then I noticed that as you emerge from the world in which your ambition is to get through the day, the trials of normal life return as well. For several months I'd forgotten I needed to get the guttering fixed. Throughout that time, even if water had cascaded down the wall to form puddles under the fuse box, I'd have thought, *I can't deal with that while I'm going through radiotherapy*, and put it out of my mind.

Sometimes I'd receive an email from a company about a missed payment or insurance renewal and it would barely register, as if it was for someone else, the person I used to be. My neighbours' pleas about the apple tree kept going unanswered.

Now I had no excuse. Once again I had to open my post. Now I had to calculate how much more the mortgage would be each month, after I'd taken six months off from the payments.

It was like having to clear up after a party, in which I'd been enjoying myself being irradiated every day with not a care in the world.

Two weeks after my treatment ended, as the body displayed spring-like symptoms of renewed life, the news channels combusted with the story that the King had cancer. 'Oh, they're ALL jumping on the bandwagon now,' I said to anyone who commented on it to me.

For the next few days every discussion that could take place was repeated many times on every news channel, almost all of them meaningless because the type of cancer hadn't even been revealed.

A year earlier I might not have noticed this detail; I'd only have known the King had cancer and that meant he would probably die from it. But now I thought that as it had been detected in its early stages, he would probably be alright after a kerfuffle, depending on what sort of cancer it was.

I was aware that cancer is an almost hopelessly vague word, covering hundreds of types of cell mutations.

But this wouldn't satisfy the demand for news, in which presenters told us solemnly, 'Welcome back to our rolling news Royal Cancer special programme; we have 40 reporters covering every aspect of the King's condition ...' You wouldn't be surprised if they said, 'Now we're going live to special reporter Sophie Buttersquash, who has a cancer-cam inside the royal sphincter.'

At one point during the extended coverage, the BBC gave us a live update that said, 'Buckingham Palace tourists say "We think he'll pull through".'

Oh, thank the Lord for that, because theirs is the opinion that matters.

I was the same when I got my diagnosis. When Dr Oikonomou told me I had a high chance of cure, I thought, *Never mind what you reckon, mate, I need to know what a Japanese bloke outside Buckingham Palace thinks.*

Then came the headlines along the lines of 'Did Meghan Markle Cause King's Cancer?', 'King's Condition is Diana's Revenge, Says Royal Medium' and 'Defence Expert Warns King's Cancer Could Be Part of Hamas Terrorist Plot'.

It was one of the moments when I felt that anti-monarchists like me are kinder towards the royals than the monarchists. Because I'm sure my experience wouldn't have been improved if I'd had hundreds of experts speculating on Sky News on how my cancer was likely to affect my public appearances.

There were some ways in which the King's status would help him. There wasn't much chance those reporters would tell us, 'The King has called the hospital and is still waiting to be put through as there's been a shortage of staff for the last five years. He called and pressed 2, then 4, then 4 again, then 3 and was put through to the maternity ward by mistake, then cut off. I'm told he shouted, "confounded ghastly system", but that is as yet unconfirmed.'

It was unlikely the newspapers would report 'King's Biopsy Lost in Transit' or 'Hope for King as Consultant Says "Touch wood".'

There was no chance he'd be driving round and round the car park looking for a space, panicking that he'd miss an appointment as he shouted, 'Why is there no room for a horse-drawn carriage in this frightful carbuncle of a building?' But cancer is a great leveller. From the earliest days of human society, certain people have been deemed to be naturally above the rest of the population because of their blood line, worthy of reverence and anointed by the gods to govern. From there all manner of medical theories have followed.

In the eleventh century there was a widespread belief that a touch from the King could cure the disease of scrofula. The lymph glands, the same little organs in which I discovered that lump, would swell as a result of this disease, but a touch from Edward the Confessor would sort it out.

This belief of royal cure spread across Europe and continued until the eighteenth century.

But eventually evidence defeated this theory, as it became apparent that not only does a monarch's touch not cure diseases, but monarchs can't stop themselves getting diseases.

The King may then be offered the finest doctors, the most rapid treatment, the Rolls-Royce of scans on a daily basis and exquisite cakes while he's being attached to his drip for the chemotherapy, but the body will go through the same discomfort as anyone else's.

Once I was hooked into my system of treatment, I can't think of many ways in which it would have been improved if I was the King. In the chemotherapy ward, there was a sign that directed private patients to the upstairs room and I wondered how that was different from the NHS chemotherapy.

Were the cannulas made from solid silver? Did the drips give off the scent of an orange grove? Were the stands the drips rested on motorised, so instead of pushing them along with you to the toilet you could ride on it, like an electric scooter? If a King had exactly the same cancer as mine, they may have a servant to prepare the steam, which

I suppose would be poured into a Wedgwood bowl first owned by George III. But the substantial part of the discomfort, the coughing and the spitting and the wheezing, would be identical.

A King won't have to worry about how his kids will manage financially if he expires, but I'm sure he'll feel the same sickening surges of anxiety as he sits in the consultant's pristine office, adorned by tropical plants, and tries to read his mood in the moments before he explains the results of the scan.

As a divinely appointed ruler, a King's status will grant him countless advantages. But as his body isn't really divine but thoroughly human, he will have to face the same nastiness that anyone with this sickness has to put up with. In some ways he will never have been further from his subjects. In other ways, maybe the King with cancer is closer to them than ever before.

*

At exactly the same time another royal intrigue developed, in which future Queen Kate Middleton disappeared from public view. Conspiracy theories multiplied as to where she might be, then she released a photo, taken several months earlier, which had been crudely photoshopped to appear current.

Newspapers shrieked with speculation and demanded to know where she was until she announced on film that she too had cancer. She'd had a course of chemotherapy, her statement said, to cure cancer in her abdomen.

I felt usurped. My daughter suggested I should have copyrighted my condition. My cancer hardly counted now two of the most prominent royals had it.

For some people, Kate's announcement didn't change a thing; they carried on demanding more revelations, presumably hoping the biopsy would be laid in a box in Westminster Hall so they could queue up and see it.

And the conspiracies continued, from people who thought the cancer story was made up to conceal something more sinister and magical. Among the evidence for this was that she couldn't have had cancer because 'she looks well'.

This was where I felt most connected to the future Queen. Her revelation came at the time when I was waiting for the scan that takes place three months after the end of the treatment. This is the one that assesses how successful, or not, it all was. By now I was presenting myself to the world as if I was back to normal, delighted to be out in public even if I felt restricted when I was there.

It's an eerie period, in which the delirium at being back out in the world is tempered by chunks of your body not working and the spectre of the scan. This is the time when so many people tell you, from a well of kindness and hope, 'It's SO good to see you've recovered and you're looking SO WELL.'

With cruelty you have to reply that while that's very sweet of them, you're recovering from the treatment but the cancer may still be burrowing away. You don't know yet as you haven't been tested.

And they say, 'But you LOOK well.'

They say it because they want you to be well. So it would be awful to respond by saying, 'Yes, but looking well doesn't mean anything because the doctor isn't going to say, "I don't think we need to bother with the scan for you because your cheeks are so rosy that your cancer has obviously gone away".'

It made me think about a night I spent with Linda when she must have been going through something similar. We travelled together with Warren to Paris for a birthday party, and she danced until two in the morning. Again I became convinced she was fine. She must have had people telling her 'You LOOK well' then too. I looked well the previous summer, when I was swimming in the south of France, four days before the doctor felt my neck and said 'hmmm'.

Anyone who has a cold with a particularly runny nose looks less well than most cancer patients on the day of their diagnosis.

At least I didn't have armies of cynics reassuring each other that as I looked well I'd obviously made the whole thing up, probably so I could take the world's gold to Bill Clinton.

It's a symbol of how the assumptions of cancer are so mistaken, that so many people believe it's incurably deadly, but also that if you look well you must have got rid of it, or never had it in the first place.

*

Another observation the princess may have made is that cancer doesn't change the people around you. If you know someone who displays their emotions openly, when they hear about your condition they will wave their arms, gasp 'Oh. My. God' and get a tear in their eye. If someone is studiously practical they will sternly give you a list of instructions and put you in touch with their sister-in-law who works for the health authority.

If someone is Christian they will say they'll pray for you; if someone responds to situations by making inappropriate jokes they'll ask if they can have the first go at sifting through your record collection if you cark it.

So the people who believe that every news statement is a lie will believe that a statement about a princess having cancer means the princess doesn't have cancer. It's quite reassuring that in so many ways, everything carries on as normal.

*

By the third week after the end of the treatment I felt a tingle of anticipation each time I woke up. What new things would I be able to do over the next few hours? Perhaps I'd be able to shout or walk up the hill to the shop and buy some Fairy Liquid. Maybe I'd drink nine sips of water or speak for five minutes on the phone without gobbing into a cup.

Every moment seemed to bring a new achievement; I felt like someone who plays violin for a symphony orchestra in the morning, wins Wimbledon in the afternoon and makes a perfect lasagne in the evening.

I still couldn't go to any social event, as spitting into a cup is frowned upon in polite society, even if it's only once every six or seven minutes. I could try telling the usher at the theatre that 'it was once every THREE minutes last week, so I'm doing well', but they might still insist I leave.

During the fourth week it occurred to me that I hadn't spat into a cup for two days so I did go to the cinema. Was this reckless? Would I be allowed to buy a ticket? Would I be asked how many times I'd spat into a cup today, by a stern manager who then told me, 'Sorry, sonny, it's against the law to let you in, I could lose my licence'? I felt delirious throughout the whole film; how could I be here?

Everywhere I went I felt like I was cheating. I'd been advised that I wouldn't be feeling 'normal' for several more weeks. But I was out at places, being social. I couldn't hear very well as my right ear was ringing, and I couldn't speak loudly. And it was all a bit exhausting and I could only drink tap water a sip at a time, but I was there, and it was beautiful.

My daughter came round with my granddaughter and we went to the park, where the toddler ran as fast as she could, while giggling and declaring, 'I'm in a RACE, Daddad' (her name for me, presumably because she's aware that 'granddad' carries social connotations of frailty and dodderiness) 'in a RACE!'

Back at the house we told the monster who lives behind the cushion to get up as he couldn't lie there all day, then she found my flossing string and unwound the whole packet until it spread majestically up and down the stairs and around everything in its path like the beams of an elaborate burglar alarm.

I went into shops and managed the whole gamut of tasks involved in buying toilet rolls and soap, then I'd hover an extra second after the purchase was complete, wanting to savour the moment.

I got stuck in a one-way system unable to find somewhere to park, turned up the music and glowed.

I bought a clock for my kitchen from a local antique shop, which I'd been meaning to do for ten years. Every part of the deal was an adventure. At every point, while deciding to buy it, as the dealer knocked the price down and as I paid for it and took it away, I was aware that three weeks earlier it would have been impossible to do any of this.

Buying a clock wasn't just a task, it was a joy. Maybe this is what some annoying spiritual preacher feels when they beam about feeling love every time they pop out for a packet of biscuits.

I'm not sure why it all felt so absurdly positive; I'd only been incapacitated for a couple of months.

I wasn't feeling happy that I was cured because there was no certainty that I had been. That assessment would be made a few months later.

Maybe it was the sense of coming out of a dark period of uncertainty. Or it was the relief of having come through an ordeal and, whatever else lay ahead, I'd finished with this episode.

But I think I felt overjoyed at every minor aspect of routine life because I had become aware of how much I missed them when they weren't there. Which is another way of saying I was confronted with how much I loved the daily and seemingly dreary tasks and interactions that fill most of our time.

An exchange with a woman in a shop about a clock is fun; it's humanly fun. Even if they're grumpy, and very few people are, the person who briefly connects with you to ask if you want a receipt, or to tell you they hope this rain stops, is adding to your sense of the society you're embroiled in.

And I'd made a decision, of whether or not to buy this clock. This was important, because I would look at this clock thousands of times. So life and its daily decisions mattered.

There was the fascination, even if absorbed unconsciously, of passing the lamps and sideboards in the shop and undergoing sensations such as 'HOW MUCH? For a fucking GLOBE!'

Every routine action was notable once I'd had it taken from my routine.

But it wasn't just that I'd missed all this; maybe it was that I'd had to confront the possibility that I wouldn't be doing any of it for much longer. And the daily routine of life was what I loved more than anything else.

One of the main motivations for wanting to live wasn't that I'd never been to Japan and hoped to go one day, or that I'd never been in a Shakespeare play and reckoned I'd be alright at it. It was the joy of undergoing the apparently irritating tasks that made up each day.

Getting round to buying a basic object after failing to do so for ten years is funny.

Listening to a track on Radio 6 Music because you

have to drive in a pointless circle is enlightening. Almost all dialogue is positive, even if it's only 'Can I put that in a bag for you?'

Whatever the reason, a wander round the shops left me less stressed and more content than it ever used to. Maybe the hospital slipped some skunk into the radiotherapy. I got home with the clock and placed it by the sink. A local odd-job man agreed to come round the next day and hang it, along with doing some other bits of hammering and drilling. In the morning, while washing up, I knocked the clock off the shelf and it smashed into so many pieces it was as if it wanted to declare, 'Don't even think you'll ever be able to mend even a bit of me.'

My son heard the clank and came into the room.

'I've broken that clock,' I said.

'It's not the end of the world,' he said.

I swept it up and poured it into the bin.

*

During the last week of my treatment, engulfed by Olympic levels of discomfort, I became capable of spotting the other end of this process. Now I was starting to consider the world beyond my immediate medical requirements.

For several months, if I'd left the house, usually it was to go to the hospital. If anyone came round, it was to see how I was and lie that I looked well.

I'd ignored any subject that might make me cross or despair. The news was dominated by the bombardment of Gaza, so I gave it no more than a fleeting glance.

One night I saw an interview with a sub-postmaster from the Post Office, one of many who had been wrongly accused of stealing money after a computer error. The story of this calm compassionate man, whose life had been battered by vicious unapologetic bureaucracy, made all my tasks seem slightly harder.

You feel helpless enough normally when you hear these stories, but it's worse when you're huddled in an immobile lump in the corner.

Somehow the process of gargling with warm water, salt and bicarbonate of soda was made more depressing by the knowledge that the government had so far refused to provide the compensation these poor sods so obviously deserved.

As I started to feel better, I could peek at it all again. During the four months of news that I'd largely avoided, it seemed that the whole of Gaza had been destroyed and a resurgent Donald Trump was on course to become president of the United States again. Couldn't I leave the rest of the world alone for a few months? Look at the state of it once I wasn't there to check up on it.

To add to the sense of global injustice, the remote control on my ridiculously over-complicated TV stopped working. I rang the shop where I bought it but they told me to ring the national helpline, which said they couldn't help. For a moment I followed my instinct, which was to tighten into a ball of anxious fury.

I felt like telling someone, 'It's UNBEARABLE, I can't even change the channel on the television, it's been ABSOLUTE HELL.'

'Stop that,' I told myself, reminding myself of my newfound stoicism and how low this all fell on the hierarchy of moaning.

And then I saw a new message from Shappi, which said, 'I'm just tiptoeing past'.

I immediately went and read back through all her messages that I hadn't seen: patient laments for my predicament and careful offers to visit. There was none of the anguish or drama or regret or hostility or concealed hostility that had infected almost every communication between us for several months before the ultrasound scan. Maybe the cancer had cured it.

Twice I'd got as far as composing a message to send to her, before changing my mind, so I stopped short of telling her everything and just thanked her for the kind thoughts and tried to explain my bodily frailties and how they'd constricted my outlook to being barely looking out at all.

She said she'd wanted to discuss Gaza with me, so I confessed that for a while I'd had no voice so I would have had to do a mime for Benjamin Netanyahu.

Fourteen

Strange Fruit

For a while, every day continued to produce a sense of liberation. There was the day when I didn't need to gargle any more. There was the day when I didn't need to put my head in steam. Then I could drink a whole glass of water in only 20 minutes, so I didn't need the syringe and feeding tube to stay hydrated.

The burning in my neck stopped so I didn't have to put cream on it. Then I had an endoscopy, at which the dieticians told me my swallowing mechanism was working almost perfectly, way ahead of schedule, so I could start eating again. I went home, where my friend Hugh gave me a poached egg on a small slice of toast, the first food I'd eaten for three months. I ate over half of it in around 40 minutes and it was one of my most memorable meals ever.

Almost the whole neck region had been blasted, including a complete obliteration of the tastebuds. I was advised there was no way of knowing how anything would taste now, so I would have to experiment.

The poached egg was noticeably an egg, more from the texture than the taste. So then I went round Sainsbury's, to wallow in the thrill of placing food in a basket.

I brought home my first bag of shopping for a while, walking past the unsteady tower of boxes of nutrition drink waiting to be syringed through the tube into my stomach. I wouldn't be needing as much of this stuff anymore, and suddenly these piles of bottles seemed like the consequence of a unique hoarding condition.

I was about to delight in the joy a baby must feel when

it first moves onto solid food, but I was 63 and in a better place to process it.

I started with a grape. I opened the packet to expose the crisp cold succulent bunch of natural sugary goodness and lovingly placed it in my mouth, like a model advertising fruit with a pornographic caress of the tongue. Within two seconds I spat it out, continuing to spit to get rid of every remaining remnant of this foul acidic bastard of a thing, making *ayagar hkkkk ohhhh ngngngng* noises as this muck flew into the sink.

There was a dull sting to this grape. In the second in which it had inflicted its damage, it had bored into every crevice, maliciously poking teeth, cheeks, throat and gums with its insipid cruelty.

For damage created in relation to size, it must have been close to a nuclear bomb. If the thing was split, the way atoms split, it could have destroyed Europe.

I had no idea that tastebuds were so subjective. I thought a grape, for example, always tasted like a grape. But it tastes like whatever our tastebuds tell it to taste like.

When Paul Hollywood frowns and laments that some poor sod on *Bake Off* has made his sauce too dry, that isn't a definitive judgement. It might be the juiciest sauce of the series but Paul's tastebuds have collapsed for the day.

Of the many questions posed by my cancer, I didn't expect that one of them would be how we knew whether anything was real.

Over the next few weeks I became familiar with the surreal nature of flavour. A tomato could taste like chicken, bacon could taste of ice cream.

If I had cheese on toast and it tasted of cheese on toast, that was probably because the toast tasted of cheese and the cheese tasted of toast.

But a bigger problem was that my saliva glands had been dug up, and you have no idea how these unsung little organs can hold the rest of us to ransom.

Who'd have thought you can't operate without moisture in the mouth? The dryness you encounter when they're not working is at a level I wouldn't have believed could exist. I've gasped through the stickiness of an arid tongue while cycling up a challenging hill on a sweltering day, eventually salivating at the oasis of a corner shop and clutching a ginger beer from their fridge. But this was nothing like that.

When your saliva glands are battered, your mouth isn't dry, it's arid, it's without any moisture at all. It feels as if a picture of your mouth would look like a photo of another planet's surface; barren, cracked and inhospitable.

Anything that went into my mouth became immediately clogged and stuck. It was like putting clay onto a potter's wheel with no water, so everything instantly becomes a crumbling stony mess.

A tiny corner of a slice of toast sucked up every droplet available like a ravenous plant, and left my tongue making an actual scraping noise as it rubbed against my mouth. Until I'd drunk half a glass of water I could only make *eyargh* sounds with no consonants like a terrible ventriloquist.

In an attempt to beat my saliva glands into submission I bought a shish kebab from the local Turkish Mezze Grill and it lasted two days. Each cube of meat had to be cut into 12 pieces and every piece had to be washed down with a whole glass of water; a close-up of a chunk falling into my stomach would have looked as if it was careering down a log flume at an Alton Towers for kebabs.

Trying to hold a conversation while eating with no saliva is a multi-tasking exercise that seems impossible, and causes social chaos.

A sliver of bread clings to your mouth so it's impossible to speak, often just as you're asked a question. So you're asked if you've got the remote control fixed for the television, but you have to reach for a glass of water, swig a mouthful to dislodge the bread, then another to prod it downwards and another to dislodge it, and all the while you can't say a word so you feel the tension, like when someone has a stutter and the other person has to wait patiently. What's the etiquette? Is it alright if they pay a parking fine or buy some cinema tickets online while they wait for you to speak?

But the most disconcerting part about the weeks of re-entry into society is that you have no idea whether any of this treatment has worked, despite the comments that it's 'so good to see you back and recovered'.

I didn't consider whether the treatment was working while I was going through it. But as I crawled out of the side-effects, a little seed of anxiety grew. At some point I would return to where all this started, in an important person's office, trying to read the way they were sitting down before they told me the results of my scan.

And if I had cancer now, that would be worse than at the beginning, because if it was still there after all this treatment it would be a highly stubborn cancer and very difficult to get rid of.

Or maybe the hospital would have a sense of nostalgia about the storyline and they could lose the results again.

*

Over the next few weeks, Shappi and I tentatively crept towards a resumption of communication. Her son and daughter spent a day with my daughter. She chose a coat for me, I read through her essay for her psychotherapy course. I told her I was failing to buy a train ticket as the website was too confusing and 'one of the advantages of having cancer is I haven't had to buy a train ticket for six months'.

She said, 'Oh, have you had cancer? You've kept that quiet.'

I replied, 'I should have been like you with your ADHD and never mentioned it.'*

She alerted me to the enigmatic podcast of a man from Limerick called *Blindboy Boatclub* and we talked about *Baby Reindeer* and her son's exams and she discovered my biological father was in London so she persuaded me to write to him.

One night, around midnight, as we were exchanging messages about our old schoolmates, after she'd discovered a boy in her class was now a professor of philosophy, she

* She mentions it quite a lot, including in a fine book, *Scatter Brain: How I finally got off the ADHD rollercoaster and became the owner of a very tidy sock drawer.*

asked suddenly, 'Did you get the *Viz* annual I sent you?'

Rarely can the mention of a *Viz* annual have stopped anyone as suddenly as it did then.

'I had no idea,' I spluttered, if you can splutter by text.

'Yes you did, you knew it was me,' she replied.

'I also sent you a Montblanc pen,' she added.

'Oh, I'm not sure I got that,' I said, panicking that I'd lost it, but not panicking as much as I would if I'd known these things cost £380.

'I was joking,' she said, 'about the pen.'

'I didn't know it was you,' I wrote, trembling a bit.

'Who else would have sent you a *Viz* annual?' she asked.

The answer was of course no one. And once again I couldn't get to sleep, but this time for different reasons from anything that had kept me awake during the previous months.

Fifteen

Suck It and See

From the time I first went to the doctor about the lump until I was told that the cancer was gone, over a year later, I didn't google any aspect of my condition.

I'm not sure if it was out of fear or distrust or laziness.

Once I felt safe, out of interest, I did. And I'm glad I'd never done it before.

If you type in 'neck cancer' or 'secondary cancer' or 'comedian from south London's metastasising cells', the results that pop up are from NHS websites, Macmillan, the UCL Cancer Institute, Wikipedia and academic-looking sites with unreadable essays full of paragraphs such as, 'Our studies of oropharyngeal cases subject to squamous carcinoma alterations (as illustrated in table 5(2ii)b fn61) suggest a steady increase of mucus development amongst bricklayers in Canada (subject to deciduous soil retention) in accordance with findings from the Hansel and Gretel Institute (Lower school, entrance behind Screwfix).'

The one quality all these websites have in common is they make anyone with the illness they're researching believe they're fucked.

For example, I read on the Macmillan Cancer Support website that if you have a primary cancer that isn't found, 'it is not usually possible to cure this cancer'.

This is fairly chilling when you have a primary cancer that wasn't found and you *have* been cured, so I'm glad I didn't see this when they first told me they hadn't found it.

If you're hunting for clues about your condition, you

will only find new ways of becoming terrified and new ways to stare at the screen muttering, 'What does that mean?'

When I mentioned to hypochondriac Matthew that I'd never at any time learned what it was exactly that I had, he replied immediately that it was something ending 'occult primary'.*

Occult primary? What the bloody hell is that? No wonder they couldn't find it if it was a poltergeist. Would my next appointment on the NHS app be to meet the dietician in the morning and then pop round to see an exorcist?

Even if you do find figures you can make sense of, does this help? Once I discovered I had a secondary neck cancer, I was assured that 'percentage survival rates for secondary neck cancer are in the nineties', which was a relief, for about three seconds. Then I thought, *Does that still leave me with a one in twelve chance of dying? In the next year? Or five years? And ninety-what? Flat ninety? Or ninety-nine?* You'd need to know as one is ten times more hopeful than the other.

When I got round to studying the internet's opinion of the cancer I'd had, I learned from the Centre for Disease Control and Prevention that 'if a patient's tumour is HPV-positive, the longterm cure rate for most stages is 80 to 90 per cent'.

So the figures I'd been given were over-optimistic. And does that statistic cover everyone? If you're a previously fit 40-year-old, are your long-term survival chances the same as someone who's 103 or a heroin addict?

* Matthew assured me the full title of my illness is metastatic squamous cell carcinoma of the neck with occult primary.

If I'd read that before the treatment had begun, I'd have scrutinised every word of that sentence. 'Longterm'? What does that mean? Long-term for a Second World War aircraft gunner is different from long-term for a newly created galaxy.

Anyone's chances of survival at any time are less than 100 per cent, especially if you're lumped in with everyone including bullfighters and people who only eat Maltesers.

To have this knowledge at a time of uncertainty could only increase your anxiety. Or it could lead to some unhelpful decisions if you calculated that the statistics showed you had a higher chance of surviving if you lived by the seaside or kept poultry.

From the moment that a plan of treatment was suggested by Dr Oikonomou, I felt an expectation from the medical team that I'd be cured, and while that couldn't be definite, I went along with that expectation.

The team of medical experts seemed to agree on a course of action, based on previous results, so I followed their suggestions as I didn't have the capacity to learn enough to dispute it with any purpose.

It's only when I consider this in retrospect that I see the value of confidence in the people who are making these decisions. All of them spoke in a relaxed tone that oozed 'expectation of cure'.

Most of what they predicted happened at the time they foresaw, they explained their analysis simply, their meetings started on time, they radiated the most valuable essence of sticking to a plan, and if they had doubts they never showed.

Of all the research you can do into someone's reliability,

nothing is as effective as an indefinable sense that someone knows what they're doing. Whenever I spoke to them, it was clear they'd read the notes made by others, they'd listened to my answers to their questions, they knew the names of everyone else who had spoken to me, they knew I was a comic, that I lived in south London, that I always said 'I'd make a terrible junkie' when the cannula didn't go in. They never stared into the middle-distance during meetings, despite this being the seventh meeting of their day.

I couldn't be certain from this that they were in any way qualified, but they *felt* as if they were, so I could do as they asked and not bother researching anything that would take me to the point of doubting them.

After I became convinced I would recover completely, I took a slight interest in what I'd been cured of, but there was one area that I was especially pleased not to have known about while the cancer was still with me. And that led me into all the googling I'd avoided up until then.

My cancer, like around 70 per cent of modern head and neck cancers, was HPV, which stands for human papillomavirus.

In the early stages of diagnosis, you want it to be HPV, because the head and neck cancer that isn't HPV comes not from a virus but from an external influence on the body, such as smoking or alcohol, and that's much more aggressive and more difficult to treat.

And over the last 40 years, as cancer from smoking has become rarer because far fewer people smoke, the proportion of HPV cancers has risen. And the cause of this, it's widely accepted, is oral sex.

The Institute of Cancer and Genomic Sciences, for example, states: 'Researchers confirmed that a higher number of lifetime oral sex partners increased the risk of HPV-related oropharyngeal cancer.'

It specifies, 'Those with six or more lifetime oral-sex partners are 8.5 times more likely to develop oropharyngeal cancer than those who do not practise oral sex.'

Honestly, you just try to be nice and look at the trouble it causes you.

This is just one report but all the others make similar findings. It turns out the virus is passed on into the mouth or throat and can sit there for many years until it's activated, like an unexploded bomb that goes off for no apparent reason after sitting under a bush since 1944.

This was compelling news. It didn't cause me any regret, because I couldn't possibly have known at the time (or indeed times), and even if I'd had an inkling, for me at the age of 27 to have said, 'I hope you don't mind but I'm not going to do that because a series of studies have suggested it makes it 8.5 times more likely that I'll develop oropharyngeal cancer,' would have entailed me being an entirely different person.

Teenage girls are now offered vaccinations against the HPV virus, which is the probable reason for a decline in the number of women who have contracted HPV-cervical cancer. So there's now a campaign, which has been largely successful, for a similar vaccination programme to be offered to boys, as the growth of HPV-head and neck cancers is fast enough for many doctors to describe as an 'epidemic'.

The arguments against such a programme seem only to be that the evidence isn't yet conclusive, or that a vaccine will 'encourage promiscuity', as if the threat of cancer is an excellent natural way of stopping teenagers from wanting sex.

And so it turns out, no matter how much I could try and shut out the outside world from my cancer, my cancer was at all times a product of and a part of the outside world.

Future research may discover the social reasons for the growth of oral sex in the late twentieth century. Maybe there will one day be a guideline as to how much is safe, as there is with alcohol. So you'll tot up your weekly units and decide not to do it again until Tuesday as it's better to be safe than sorry.

And in the meantime the battle will rage, not just within science but between science and those who are hostile to science, as it interferes with the wholesome rules that came from outside humanity altogether.

From the medieval priesthood that opposed the experimenting on corpses by physicians as it 'spoiled God's work', to the politicians of the 1980s who insisted the way to deal with AIDS was to tell people not to be so gay, medicine has had to counter superstition.

I should have anticipated that my cancer would want to be part of that battle.

Sixteen

One Better Day

In the early days of my cancer scare, I'd arrogantly wondered whether, if I died, my death would be noted at Crystal Palace Football Club. There's a tradition – established recently – that the passing of certain fans is commemorated by a mass round of applause at the minute in the game that corresponds with the age of the deceased. So if the fan was 54, the applause happens during the 54th minute.

So the disaster, if you want to be remembered like that, would be to live longer than 90 because the game only lasts 90 minutes. Expiring in my mid-sixties would give me a chance of a memorial applause, which would be quite a consolation, I thought. Over the next few weeks I crept back towards normality. I bought tickets for Crystal Palace's home match against Burnley, cautious about being in a crowd while I couldn't speak properly, or hear properly, or eat or drink, hadn't walked more than a few yards for several months, felt dizzy when I stood up and my favourite subject of conversation was how I couldn't produce any saliva.

It was an important game for Palace, as defeat would leave them in danger of relegation, but my internal commentary was going, *This is a vital fixture, that will determine whether Mark can keep up with the elite who can go out and watch things. WHAT a contest it's going to be.*

At the game, several people shook my hand, patted me on the back and said it was great to see me, then asked how I was. I croaked that I was recovering and excited to be out but couldn't speak much, then they would ask me to tell them all about it but could I speak up a bit.

Several people offered to buy me a beer. One of them was already at the bar, so I said, 'I'd love a sip of tap water.'

'Water?' he bellowed. 'You deserve a beer after what you've been through!' He pulled a face that said, *Blimey, I knew cancer was bad but I didn't realise it stopped you having a pint before the football.*

It was a beautiful two hours, a tentative re-entry into a world where thousands of people scream, berate, fume and cheer irrationally, and in between these displays of emotion, some of them would squat next to me and say, 'Glad to see you looking well, Mark.'

For each of these people, it would have been easier to note from a distance, if they were interested, that although they'd heard from somewhere or other that I had cancer, I'd made it to a football match. Instead they went out of their way to let me know they were pleased about this.

At half-time in a football ground, conducting a conversation is a battle upstream against the guttural statements of the 1,000 men and 20 women in your area, sporadic outbursts of song and people barging into your back with one more flimsy plastic cup of lager than they can carry. It's an impossible challenge and it's even trickier when you're recovering from radiotherapy.

People offered me chips, told me jokes lost in the echoey buzz pinging through my irradiated ears and asked what sort of chemo I'd had. It was my introduction to an inspirational experience of mass kindness that's so generous it could be annoying.

'You look so well,' they'd roar with an operatic flourish, arms out wide.

'Thanks, I'm on the mend,' I'd squeak, but might as well have mimed it as the husky words barely dribbled past my lips.

It was only nine months since I'd last been there, but it all seemed slightly distant. Is this really what I used to do? It was another routine that, having stopped doing it for a while, I was compelled to re-examine why I bothered doing it.

Maybe everyone should have to take nine months off their normal routine, to give them a chance to reconsider whether there's any point to it.

Priests would come back after their nine months and think, *What the bloody hell do I do this for every Sunday? I mean, there's not even any actual evidence he exists.*

Blokes who have been to the same pub with the same lads every Thursday for 15 years would realise they don't enjoy it very much, and wouldn't go back until one of them has a new anecdote.

But I did love this pointless carnival: singing 'Glad All Over' as the team comes out, the crowd rising as one to howl 'yer dirty bastard' when your player's fouled, the energy, the noise, the emotion, the outbreaks of song, the joyful collective spirit of 25,000 people playing their role (the shouty ones, the sullen ones, the adversarial away fans, the nerdy ones, the furious ones) to create a ridiculous piece of improvised theatre. Rather than turn up out of habit, I'd been forced to re-evaluate whether I wanted to be part of it and decided I did, which made it more beautiful than ever. The result of the match barely mattered.*

Later in the week I tried a party, a friend's book launch, which was unlikely to be quite as noisy. I met my friend Angela outside and walked in, just like that, as if I was normal.

But this was much more difficult, because at the football there were two periods of 45 minutes when I could sit and say nothing. Here I was expected to speak. 'Brilliant to see you, I didn't expect to see you at anything like this for a while,' said several people.

'How are you? You LOOK well,' they said.

Lots of people offered me a beer. 'A glass of tap water, please,' I'd say, squeakily.

'Water? You want something more than water, don't you? After all you've been through,' said the first person.

My mouth was so dry I couldn't move any of the parts needed to make a word.

'Orter,' I grunted, like a neanderthal that had been discovered in the woods and was being taught language for the first time.

Then the barman asked if I wanted still or sparkling, with ice or lemon or lime and if so, fresh lemon or cordial, and a pint or a half.

Even a grunted word was beyond me now, so I said 'ng'.

So he went through all the options again and a new person arrived to ask how I was and I pointed to the barman who was stood waiting for his answers, so I mimed a tap being turned on and maybe he wondered whether that was sign language for lime cordial and I wished I was

* It was Crystal Palace 3, Burnley 0.

in the twelfth century because you would just arrive at a well and get the one water there was, which was probably full of cholera but at least there wouldn't be all this fuss.

After a few delicate sips, I could speak quietly but then the food arrived, a magnificent display of pub party-food: pork pies and chicken wings and tiny sausages and mustard. I took a sausage and nibbled a sliver – the amount you find stuck in your teeth as you're going to bed.

More people asked how I was, so I chewed and chewed and swallowed and washed down my ladybird-sized whisper of sausage and puffed, 'I'm fine, thank you, but talking and eating are difficult.'

And they all smiled and said they'd leave me to my sausage, except one man who said, 'So what type of cancer was it then?'

By now I'd taken on another sliver so I chewed some more, a bit flustered as he was waiting for an answer, until I wheezed, 'Round the throat area. Sorry, it's really hard to talk or eat.'

'Are you doing another series of going round the towns?' he asked. At least I could nod to this.

'Which ones are you doing, Mark? My wife loves them shows, more than I do, to be honest. Which places are you going to?'

I gestured that this may take a while. I chewed and chewed and took some water, all the while feeling like when someone has asked you a question and you're waiting for a slow computer to upload so you can give them an answer.

'Margate,' I said.

'Where? You'll have to speak up, there's a right racket in here.'

'Marhat,' I said, then had to have some water.

'Margate? Oh, Margate, what did you make of that?'

I mimed a sort of 'so-so' gesture.

'What's Dreamland like these days? Here, I'll get my wife, she's only just over there, she loves those shows, she'll have so much to ask you.'

'Hard to talk,' I said, as if I was auditioning to play the Elephant Man.

'Alright, Margate, where else?' he said.

'Sorry, I need concentrate sosk.'

'On what?'

'Soskage.'

'Oh yeah, that's giving you trouble, is it? Here, try a pork pie. Have you ever thought about doing Ipswich?'

Eventually I found a corner where I could sit with my back to the room and give this party sausage, the size of a large Cheesy Wotsit, the attention it demanded. After about 30 minutes, I got the bastard down.

People who I had seen regularly throughout many years, but for the last nine months had existed as a couple of text messages read between inhalations of steam, smiled and told me I looked well and asked if I was going on holiday or what I thought about Gaza and I'd tell them it was hard to speak and someone handed me a pint of Guinness and everyone was so wholesomely kind that I longed for a room of rude people so I could sit and rest and I shuffled out of the door and went home.

*

Most messages and appointments from the hospital were conveyed by email or text, which popped up on my phone, any time, sitting there waiting to be opened like a box on *Deal or No Deal*. Sometimes I would plunge straight in and open it like an all-year open swimmer diving into an icy pond. Other times I would leave it festering away, waiting for the right time to peek at it to find out whether I'd get to August.

The NHS understands the rules of drama, so you can't simply click on the message and read it. You have to sign in with an email and username, then you're sent a code which you enter into a box and then you can find out which appointment you have or the results of a test on some internal organ or other.

One day the message told me that after my meeting with the dietician the next day, I was to meet the whole team dealing with me, including the consultant. I'd only met the whole team once before so this must be serious.

What could they have discovered? I hadn't had any tests recently, so had they become convinced the cancer was spreading from the way I was walking?

Another message arrived to confirm the appointment, so I tried all the techniques we use to stay calm. There could be many reasons for this sudden meeting: it could be a routine check-up they'd forgotten to tell me about, I could have won a prize for being the millionth cancer patient in Britain, they might all want to know which towns I was going to for the next radio series.

So I relaxed into a state of suppressed anxiety, in which the body is clamouring to be a sweaty worried whirlpool but the head is telling it to relax so they reach a compromise of a dull worry that rests somewhere between stomach and bowels.

After I'd seen the dietician, I forced the anxious fireworks away and approached the reception, where you wait to be called into a room with a consultant. The mundanity of these meetings never stops being remarkable. A receptionist takes your name in exactly the tone used by the bored woman in the dry cleaner's when you've come to pick up a jacket. You prepare to be asked to sit down and wait, with the intonation the announcers use in the Co-op to remind you there's a special three-for-two offer on Greek yoghurt. 'Take a seat until you're called in to be told if you'll live or die. Toilets are on the left at the back of the reception area.'

But this time she looked at her screen, slightly quizzically. What could this mean? Had they mixed me up with another Mark Steel, who died from pleurisy in 1894? 'Oh, sorry, Mark,' she said, 'there's no appointment today, the system sent this out by mistake. It does that sometimes.'

*

Sometimes the messages would arrive in the night, so I'd see one as I woke up and through the mist of the day's first moments I'd clumsily try to tap in codes and remember passwords.

What might it tell me, this nocturnal automatically sent note on an iPhone? Sometimes they contained a result from a blood test that I'd forgotten about. Maybe it revealed a higher-than-expected platelets per mcl figure. What did this mean? It was 6.15 in the morning and I was panicking about safe levels of platelets per mcl. Instead of this iciness, shouldn't these messages and results come with a human flourish, such as, 'These look bad but it can go like this if you've had a banana so it's probably fuck-all.'

One day it told me with digital diffidence that I would have my post-treatment MRI scan on 11 April, to see whether all the activities of the last nine months had succeeded.

The advice for dealing with an impending moment like this, which determines the rest of your life or even how much of a rest of your life there is, goes 'put it out of your mind'. But that's impossible. You can put it out of the front of your mind but it's always there, lurking like a patch of mould on the ceiling. You can get on with other thoughts but you'll only add to your stress if you pretend it isn't there at all. The effects of the treatment were receding. Gradually the tastebuds recognised stronger sensations: I developed a craving for crisps, tomatoes tasted like battery acid and in a glorious moment I consumed a sip of Guinness. Anything vaguely sweet – chocolate, cake, a bun or lemonade – tasted evil. It wasn't just unpleasant; sweetness was a deliberately malicious flavour created by far-right terrorists out of spite. I went to the gym, went cycling, recorded an episode of my radio show in Margate, drinking three pints of water through the show, which must be the amount of saliva I usually get through.

One morning I felt a strange globular stickiness that skipped across the tongue like a goose flitting over a lake.

It was at an unexpected moment and a couple of minutes later I wondered if it had been a droplet of saliva, a beautiful golden ball of spit, that if it had been filmed would have been surrounded by a dazzling aura. I couldn't be certain, but it felt like a symbol of a new era, like the first crocus of spring. If I'd been alert to it, when it happened I would have dribbled it out and kept it in a velvet box.

Eventually I could devour a slice of toast in 15 minutes. Often I relied on soup, and I became fearful of horrors such as lettuce, which would cling to the throat, refusing to descend, like someone grasping a tree branch on the side of a cliff.

Chicken was manageable but I had to cut it into minuscule portions so anyone watching would think I was taking it home for a recovering hedgehog. Eggs slid down joyfully, rice was a disaster, muesli needed two pints of milk per spoonful.

In a pub I ordered pie and mash, an act of bravado as arrogant as when Al Pacino's blind character drives a car. It took around two hours and six jugs of gravy that the waiter must have suspected I was smuggling to somewhere in the Middle East where gravy is illegal.

Any time I went to a cafe I would ask for a pint of water. Sometimes they only dealt out small dainty glasses, so I'd have to go back every two or three minutes and ask for more.

When I told all this to a dietician at a hospital appointment, she said, 'It must be very frustrating.'

I let out an involuntary shriek of 'NO.'

'A few months ago,' I said, 'I was feeding myself through

a tube. I couldn't even imagine drinking a cup of coffee or slowly sucking on a sliver of water-assisted chicken. You people saved my life. I can't tell you how inconsequential it is to be unable to have a chocolate Hobnob or to need a bucket of gravy to eat a pie.' She made a note and asked if I could manage a whole banana.

My physical life was easing back to normal, except for one detail – there was no guarantee I didn't still have cancer. It was possible I would still face a moment, perched on the edge of a chair in an office opposite a consultant with a sympathetic smile who would say, 'It's not gone as well as we hoped.'

A couple of months after the treatment had ended, it was normal for people to approach me in shops and tell me they were so pleased I had come through it all. Sometimes they'd ask if I was definitely clear and I'd say I hadn't yet had the scan. 'I'm sure you'll be fine,' they'd say.

This could only have been reassuring if they worked in the hospital and had seen my private notes, but it was always heartening because it was their way of saying they *wanted* me to be fine.

There's a strange psychological quirk in asking someone how they are, if the answer may be seriously in question. We want them to be alright, mostly because we care for them but also because if they reply that they're really ill, that spoils our day as well. I met the beautifully endearing comic Phil Jerrod, who died of cancer in 2021 at the age of 42, at an open-air theatre in Brighton where I was performing, when his illness had bolted him into a wheelchair.

We talked a bit about shows we'd seen and about shows he'd been part of and he said, 'I'm pretty much finished with that now,' as breezily as if the reason he'd stopped performing was that he'd taken up dog-grooming instead.

I knew his illness was incurable, but when he said, 'They're just managing me until the end now,' I must have conveyed an undisguised cocktail of shock and sadness so he said, 'Oh, sorry, I didn't want to be miserable.'

For a moment his thought process was *Sorry I'm dying*, which is criminally absurd.

But the terrible truth is that a natural part of the human reaction *is* to be disappointed that the other person has spoiled our mood. There's a primeval urge to say, 'Oh, thank you VERY much for bringing us all down. We were having a jolly chat in the sunshine until you brought impending death into it.'

When a friend, acquaintance or stranger told me I looked well, they wanted me to be well. They didn't want their mood jolted because my outward demeanour was no guide to whether potentially errant cells were still misbehaving around my lymph nodes.

I had a social responsibility to be completely cured.

*

I went to Malvern in Worcestershire to absorb as much as I could about the town so I could write a radio show about it. One of the purposes of Malvern is to be ridiculously hilly, so it was a slight struggle walking around but it was a hypnotically effusive day.

It started when a local man from the theatre told me, 'A wonderful thing about Malvern is the Cotswolds are in the way of it, which is handy as it stops people coming from London. It means if they want to come here, they either have to see Birmingham or Swindon and that puts them off.'

It's the sort of proud grumpiness that ignites these shows, and my producer Carl and I started giggling as we usually do on these trips.

We went up to the beacon and round an iconic church and to local hero Edward Elgar's grave and had lunch in a cafe full of leaflets advertising local Pilates groups, because I reckoned I could manage their lentil soup.

It was my favourite sort of day, which I've cherished since first making these programmes: a day I didn't dare imagine three months earlier as I took a rest every two steps after a morning's radiotherapy.

In the evening I sat in the car to drive home, and a text pinged that I decided to glance at before I set off.

It came from my cancer buddy Jules, who had been to a meeting about his scan results. The treatment had slowed down his cancer, he'd been told, but hadn't removed it. This was an aggressive swine of a cancer, and it couldn't now be cured.

There were methods of containing it, he said, and the daft irony of the situation was he felt tremendously fit, had been exercising and rowing and everyone he met told him 'you LOOK well'.

But while he would remain positive, he said, 'It appears I'll have to retire hurt before I've finished my innings.'

I felt the dull tingle of despairing reality that sucks in your stomach and face and makes you unable to move or speak for a while, as your mind searches for hope but needs to be told to stop looking.

I felt so bad for Jules and his family, but also it was a reminder that my story was far from over, and then I felt disgusted with myself for responding to this message by thinking about how it related to me.

This was the situation we all fear, where an expert who you only recently met sits before you to explain that the life story you imagined for yourself will be cut abruptly short, and you'd best prepare for it.

The basic idea of the Stoics, that you must fight to improve what you can alter but must accept what you can't, is put to its ultimate test in a moment like this. This is European Champions League stoicism.

I, on the other hand, replied with a message to say sometimes a batter can retire hurt but come back later in the innings, and then I drove home feeling very inadequate.

*

The process of the MRI scan itself is impressively mundane. I arrived on my own, where a nurse asked if I had a preferred vein for the cannula. *Ah, this takes me back*, I thought.

So we went through the old routine. 'You might need a specialist nurse – I'm sure it will be fine – this might sting a bit – humph – oh – OK just a bit of a sting here – *phhhhhhhhh* – one more try – *aahhhhh phoo*, I'll see if one of the other doctors can help.'

Then you're shown a locker where you put your keys, and you sign a series of forms to declare you have nothing metallic on you that will send the powerful magnets that drive the scanner doolally. I wonder how often patients forget they have an earring, so the scan starts and they're suddenly twirled into a somersault and find themselves clinging upside-down to the wall as if they're being sucked out of a plane.

Then you get rolled into a tube for 25 minutes, then rolled out again like a car mechanic that's been poking at a chassis.

'There are your shoes, you'll get the result in a few weeks, don't forget your hat,' the nurse told me before going into her office. I collected my things and thought, *I can't go, just like that, after a scan that will determine whether I've still got cancer.* So I opened the door of an office and said, 'Bye, then,' to everyone in there.

'Yes, bye,' said one of them without looking up from the form they were filling in. And I left. I know the NHS struggles for funding, but shouldn't there be a cake and fireworks?

The meeting to discuss the results had been scheduled on the app for three weeks later. But I was due to meet a consultant two weeks before that, to discuss how I was recovering from the effects of the treatment. On the way to the hospital I became convinced they would have the results already and I would find out that afternoon if I was cancer-free. For the first time ever, the appointment was delayed.

I sat in reception trying to read a book, but every line bounced back at me with my mind complaining, *I can't take this in now.*

I considered buying a bag of crisps, wondering how this might affect my anxiety. I could feel the sweat forming a sticky puddle under each arm and went to the toilet to wash it away, worrying I'd be called and miss the appointment and out of spite they wouldn't tell me the results.

One hour late I was called in, where the charming consultant beamed a big hello, as if we were simply meeting to pop out for a curry. He said, 'I did ask if your results were through but they haven't been processed yet,' as if they were a minor detail, less important than whether I'd noticed he had a new plant on his desk. 'Anyway, how do you feel? You LOOK well.'

All the glands and neurones and parts of the heart that deal with anxiety stood down. 'False alarm, results not in yet,' they called out, and I was aware I'd been sweating under the armpits for nothing.

'That's fine,' I said, 'I'm sure they'll be through soon.'

And I wanted to lie sprawled across the table like a fainting maiden in a Victorian drama, gasping, 'When, when will we get them? Spare me such heartache.'

'Oh, I'm sure they'll be alright when we get them,' he said.

A few days later, one week before the rescheduled results meeting, I was called by an assistant who said I didn't need to come in at all, I would be told the results by phone on the Tuesday at 10am.

What could that mean? Surely this suggested the results were good. They wouldn't tell me bad news by phone, would they? 'Sorry, but your cancer has gone all over the place. It's so rampant that we had to bring the discussion forward a day as we're not sure you'll make it to tomorrow.'

The power of the unknown result increased with each day, despite me trying to write a show about East Grinstead for the *In Town* series.

I spent the days before the results announcement writing the script, talking to the producer and reading about the town. I nonchalantly referred in conversation to something that would happen in 'two weeks' time' or 'next Wednesday', but this always gave me a jolt, a reminder there would come a time when I knew whether all the mucus, the time under the mask, the cannulas, the operation, the tubes, the steam, the biopsies, the chemo and the touching of wood had worked.

I asked my son to make sure he would be with me at 10am. I arranged a list in my head of people to call after I'd heard from them. And I ran through the probable way the call would start, in my mind, so I wouldn't be too flustered when it happened.

I guessed there would be a moment when I would be asked, 'How are you today?' And I planned that I would say I was feeling fine but 'you know better than me how I am in the long run, because you've got my results in front of you'.

I guessed there would be a preamble, during which time I'd feel like shouting, 'Never mind all this, tell me whether or not the fucking cancer's gone.'

I guessed the call would be late, so 10 o'clock would pass and maybe some people would call to ask how it went before I'd been told, then the phone would ring and I'd answer with a scurried fumble but it would be someone from EE telling me about an exciting new contract they could offer me on my next phone upgrade.

I ran through the possible scenarios, which they'd suggested would be one of three possibilities: that the cancer had gone completely, that it hadn't gone entirely but was still receding so the treatment was still working and we'd have to wait a few months before knowing for certain, or that there was still cancer in my body so I would need further treatment.

I prepared myself for each one so I'd react calmly and ask the questions that would be most useful, I made myself familiar with the thoughts that might swirl around me in the moment and I did all this while being very careful to put the awaited phone call out of my mind.*

*

The day before the call I had to go for an appointment about the imbalance that had been created in my lymphatic system.

The Slovakian doctor examined me to check on the build-up of lymphatic fluid that results from radiotherapy.

She unfurled a life-size diagram of a body with the lymphatic system displayed, a baffling diagram of loops,

* I was particularly fascinated by East Grinstead because it's a town of around 25,000 people in West Sussex, just outside the M25, quiet, suburban, containing only the facilities you'd expect: a library, a theatre, a branch of Caffè Nero, the second biggest Mormon church in Britain and a 100-acre manor housing the headquarters of European Scientology, where Tom Cruise stays regularly and John Travolta once provoked a front page in the local paper when he tried to reserve a table for four at the local Kentucky Fried Chicken.

squiggles and tributaries, like a map of the rivers and streams of Canada.

With dazzling enthusiasm she explained that this system of fluids flows around the body, containing elements that battle bacteria. But there is also a complex series of 'nodes' that act like locks in a canal system, regulating the fluid so it disperses evenly.

My first thought was that the creationists must be right. How could such elaborate engineering be caused by evolution?

Becoming a fundamentalist Christian adhering to the literal texts of the Bible might take my mind off the next day's phone call.

The nodes around my neck, like everything else in that region, had been battered by the radiotherapy. If they weren't operating, the fluid would gush from the neck to collect under my chin, creating a ball of fluid that hung down as if I was a pelican.

Who could have guessed there are so many moving parts to the human body? I'd never even heard of this system until I had cancer there. What other hidden mechanisms have we got? Is there one that puffs out a pungent aroma from the back of our knees that's undetectable by other humans but is repellent to owls and stops them from eating us in the night?

Her tests revealed I had much less damage to my lymph nodes than expected, which I should have been delighted about but it all seemed so trivial compared to whether the cancer had gone or not. If I found out the next day that the cancer was still spreading, I suppose at least I could be confident that I'd die with my lymph nodes in reasonable condition.

That evening I exchanged some messages with Shappi about Gestalt psychotherapy and sat on my own watching *The Equalizer*, a Denzel Washington film in which he kills dozens of people with barely a thought. What could be more relaxing in these circumstances than a film about the routine nature of death?

The next morning, on a crisp clear April day, I started writing at about seven and was strangely productive. Apart from an optimistic message from Shappi and a letter about a parking fine, there was no communication with anyone.

At 9.30, the phone rang. It wouldn't be the hospital; they wouldn't call 30 minutes before they'd said they would.

'Hello, is that Mr Steel?' said a voice I didn't recognise.

'Yes, that's me,' I said as cheerily as I could.

'I'm calling from University College Hospital,' said the man, who had the reassuring tone of a modern vicar talking to teenagers about how the church could help with their skateboard park.

'Oh, hello,' I said, trying to sound as if I'd forgotten all about this call and didn't really have time to discuss trivia such as my lifespan.

'How are you today?' he said.

Ha, I got that right, I thought.

'I've been feeling fine and everybody says I look well, I know that isn't an indicator but it feels hopeful and it's still difficult to eat because the saliva glands got damaged by the radiotherapy though I'm sure you know that as you're from the hospital and my hearings's not good but

I had a good meeting yesterday about the lymph nodes, what an extraordinary system that is, enough to make me a creationist, not really, I'm a big fan of Darwin, though you must know better than me how I am in the long run, because you've got my results in front of you.'

'Yes,' he said with compassionate authority. 'The saliva glands will repair somewhat, though some long-term damage is to be expected and the same goes for the hearing. I gather your swallowing returned much quicker than expected, which is excellent ...'

Never mind all this, I thought, *tell me whether or not the fucking cancer's gone.*

'I can tell you the scan results show you have responded to treatment.'

In the period of a quarter of a second between the end of that sentence and the start of the next, I thought, *This sounds brilliant, but hang on, I may have responded to treatment but not as much as they hoped, or what if he says next, 'Unfortunately you've responded to treatment in the wrong way so your kidneys have disappeared altogether and you've developed gills like a fish.* He went on: 'The results show no sign of disease.'

'So the cancer's gone?' I asked.

'Yes, there's no sign of cancer on the scan.'

'OK,' I said, 'I might need a moment just to take that in.'

'Of course,' he said, 'take your time. We want to look at you regularly, the routine is to check every three months for the next five years.'

Then he said some other things, about how important it was to keep using the cream on the burned areas and to get my hearing checked, but by now my emotions were slumped into a massive soft soppy armchair.

I shouted upstairs to my son and I sent Shappi the simplest message, 'The cancer's gone.'

I called my wonderful friend Matthew and my son came into the room. I said nothing and gave him a hug. I wonder how different that hug was to the one outside the hospital after I'd been told, 'It's not good news, Mr Steel.'

I left a message for my daughter, who was at work. And Shappi asked me to call her, so I did and she burst into tears, at which point it seemed probable we'd spend the rest of our lives, of which mine could now be assumed to last a fair bit longer, together (touch wood). It had been quite an emotional five minutes.

I told friends in the order I'd worked out, including Matt Forde, who called immediately and shrieked with selfless excitement, though I wish I could say he'd shrieked in the voice of Donald Trump.

I told Jules, who was exultant, and of course stoic.

I went to a friend's house as I'd promised and we all hugged and they made me a cup of tea and we watched the snooker.

It would be a while before I could figure out what I'd learned from all this. But I knew at that moment that I really enjoyed living.

Seventeen

Mortal Man

Just as the radiotherapy blasted away but couldn't be felt until the effects made themselves clear much later, so did the impact of the moment at which the doctor in Croydon answered my question about the possibility of death by saying 'touch wood'.

I'd been aware for some time that I was mortal. When I asked the question about whether my condition was likely to be fatal, I must have been very aware I was mortal. But even then I'm not sure I'd felt mortal.

Coming out of the treatment and facing the scan that would show how far I'd advanced towards a cure, I realised I now thought differently, with a sense that the future would eventually carry on without me. It was just a question of when.

This wasn't a morbid or negative thought. Maybe it was similar to an athlete accepting in their thirties that the next Olympics will probably be the last they can compete in.

Without realising it, I'd become accustomed to thinking about ten years' time being a place I may not get to. There was a high likelihood I'd be cured but a real possibility I wouldn't be.

I did a routine when I turned 50, about how at that age everything became finite. 'How many foreign holidays did I have left? Twenty-five? If I was lucky. And the last ten of those I wouldn't be aware of which country I was in. If I'm buying a book, I think, *That's way too big, it's too late to start that and have a chance of finishing it.* And even bananas: at two a week I'm down to my last three thousand.'

But now I made decisions with that mode of thinking. Each series of *In Town* takes several months to make. So if I did a few more series, that could take up a fair percentage of my remaining time even if I carried on living for another 25 years.

One of the reasons why this isn't a negative process is it can make you appreciate what you felt was familiar and mundane. I'd reaffirmed in my head that I wanted to carry on making those shows. It wasn't out of necessity or routine; I had calculated that it was still the best way I could think of to spend that time, like a couple renewing wedding vows after 20 years.

Similarly, I wanted to see more of the people who I saw anyway. There was no one about whom I felt, *Now I consider that time may be short, I'm not going to waste any of it on that boring arse.*

But I did find myself quicker to leave situations that I didn't want to be in. I noticed I was able to (politely, I hope) say I had to go, whereas before I would have stayed longer than I wished to, as it would feel a bit rude to leave. I'm sure that was a result of a clock in the back of my mind beeping that there wasn't enough time left to muck about like this. It makes sense that you cut out those moments as time gets shorter. If you were told you had 40 minutes to live, you'd have to be very weak-willed to spend 30 of them with a group of people you didn't get along with because you were worried about hurting their feelings if you left when it was only ten past nine. More poignantly, I could visualise this point in the future that I wouldn't be part of, in the way that sports players are trained to 'visualise', for example by imagining that they're serving for the match in a Wimbledon final so it's not such a nervy shock if it happens.

I could picture my son and daughter and granddaughter marching on without me and this was a joyful image, more optimistic than telling myself not to think of such things because it was too unimaginable.

Then the ego started to play a part. By the time I had the call to say 'there is no sign of disease', my granddaughter was two and a half. By now we'd agreed on an elaborate set of monsters, including one that lived under the cushion and a 'drunk' monster that always demanded beer, as well as the constantly hungry shark. (These were more creatures from her mother's era that didn't seem to have dated. I didn't have to write any new stuff at all.)

She knew me enough to shout 'Dad-dad' excitedly when I popped up on a repeat of *Celebrity Chase* one afternoon.

But however cuddly and bouncy you are with a grandchild, they won't recall anything of you if you drop dead when they're two and a half. I had this awful image of her at the age of 15, with my daughter asking her, 'You don't remember Granddad, do you? He used to pretend to be a shark and you'd shout, "Stop eating everything, you naughty shark".'

And she'd go, 'Dur, of COURSE I don't remember, I was, like, one or something.' Sod that.

I wanted to be present long enough that she would always be able to recount our days out, our jokes and conversations. I needed to stay alive for at least another ten years.

That way, with a bit of luck, I would be talked about into the twenty-second century.

*

Maybe the most cheerful and optimistic sentiment I've accepted since experiencing this illness is that we're all terminally ill, it's just a matter of how much.

We try so hard to pretend we're immortal.

There's a vague awareness, as we get older, that we might not be around for ever. At 55, you think back 30 years and it seems so appallingly recent, then it crosses your mind that the same length of time forward takes you to 85.

Then you put it out of your mind, or think about David Attenborough still making wildlife films at 95, and carry on ignoring it.

When I was 60, I saw Bruce Springsteen performing a three-hour show with unfathomable energy when he was 72 and consoled myself I'd be able to do the same, so I didn't need to worry about age for at least another 50 years.

Maybe you make a will, and discuss with your kids what will take place 'in case anything happens to me', the subtext being 'it won't but it's best to be ridiculously cautious and make allowances for the unlikely scenario that one day I'm one of those unlucky people who gets to a certain age and dies'.

We go to such lengths to avoid contemplating the end. We create an afterlife, in which our loved ones are looking down on us, as if they've just nipped away for a while, and we make barely any effort to consider how this place operates.

If we had a parent who was constantly embittered and negative, are they reprogrammed in heaven to be supportive to their kids, or are they looking down at their daughter playing the violin and going, 'I don't call that music! I'm glad I never wasted money on lessons if that's the racket you make.'

Or as Bart Simpson asked his Sunday school teacher, 'What if you're a really good person but you're in a really, really bad fight and your leg gets gangrene and it has to be amputated? Will it be waiting for you in heaven?'

The very rich might become obsessed with freezing their brains so they can be reignited when the technology advances, enabling them to enjoy a whole new existence as a paralysed series of thoughts in a world where everyone they ever knew who wasn't a billionaire is dead.

We do all this to avoid the awful probability that when we die, that is the end of our life.

For a few weeks in the summer of 2023 I had to consider the possibility that I had a disease that would kill me.

This wasn't being overdramatic, like people who say, 'I could have been killed,' when a wheelie bin blows across the road near them in a strong wind.

Or when there's news of an explosion in Nigeria and someone says, 'I was in Africa five years ago, so I realised, "That could have been me."'

I'm not sure what my odds of survival were in those early days. I reckon that on the day I discovered the lump,

Paddy Power would have offered odds of around 80/1 that it would be deadly. After I'd had the ultrasound scan, they may have cut that to 20/1. Once the tests came back suggesting cancer, I was probably 5/1, possibly shortening to 3/1 or 5/2 after the 'touch wood' moment. Maybe some punters would have been adventurous and had me on a double with Matt Forde.

Whatever the chances of it being terminal, it was strong enough for me to wonder how I would address impending death and how I could ensure the minimum palaver for my offspring.

This period of uncertainty was brief but invasive. I could feel the gravity of the situation in my organs and bones. I had always known I would die but not actually die, the way dead people have done.

The death I knew about was theoretical. It wouldn't really happen. I'd talked about the music I would have at my funeral and wondered what the world would be like in the year 3000, aware I wouldn't be in it. I'd got the forms to fill out a will and then lost them. But that's not the same as actually facing up to your real, actual death.

Now there was a deep solid weight of acceptance, swirling slowly in the stomach but reaching out to tell the rest of the body every few minutes 'this really could be it', with all that would entail, before hesitantly assuring itself not to be so daft and then creeping back to a doomful whirlpool of slurry again.

The period of facing up to this new situation evaporated after I was told that the cancer hadn't spread and I could go back to death being hypothetical.

But nine months later, when I was getting used to being cancer-free, I gradually became aware of feeling subtly, disconcertingly different. There had been no spiritual conversions, or pledges to become a fruitarian or take up pole-vaulting. I wasn't living in the woods and screaming about Jesus.

Instead there was the imprecise sensation of something unfamiliar, like the early stirrings of a character in a science fiction film who was exposed to radiation nine months earlier and feels alright now but is starting to behave out of character. (This usually ends with him running naked through the city and living on top of a mobile phone mast, buzzing like a wasp.)

Shappi said I was less frenetic, more likely to stop what I was doing to chat and wouldn't fret any more about doing as many shows as possible or piling up a working schedule guaranteed to cause a pile of stress.

She said I was less bothered about 'performing' in social situations, more 'accepting' of conditions without railing against them. The shorthand for this was that I was happier.

(The other implication is that before the cancer I must have been a right pain in the arse.)

Maybe when an anaesthetist is about to gas you or a tube is being lowered into your stomach via your nose, you learn to accept and appreciate other situations that you can't change as well.

You abandon the futile agitation that things should be different, that you should be living somewhere else, that there should be more people in your audience, the rubbish truck shouldn't be blocking the road and holding you up for two minutes or it should stop raining on a day you're supposed to be playing cricket.

One of the hardest lessons we learn as a toddler is that we can't always get what we want. I saw a frazzled dad one evening, trying to explain to his three-year-old son that he couldn't have the biscuit he wanted because the shops were shut. The boy yelled and yelled, 'But I WANT THAT BISCUIT!' and the dad asked if I had any of these particular biscuits, then knocked at his neighbour's door to ask about the biscuit and I wondered if he would end up carrying out the world's first biscuit heist at Sainsbury's. If I'd been through my cancer experience at the time, I might have been able to explain to the child the virtue of accepting that 'there are no biscuits'.

Similarly, if there are ten things you 'have to do' in a day, you screech round corners in the car and run through the house knocking things over, creating extra things to do tomorrow because now you need a new television. You ignore friends and partners because you don't have time for them and enjoy none of the ten things because you're panicking that you're late for the seventh one.

I had spent years like that, but now I'll only do three of those things, because it simply isn't possible to do more properly, or enjoyably, so I'll tell seven people I didn't have time to do their thing today, then never commit myself to such a stupid schedule again in the first place.

I also discovered the glory of enjoying a sense of achievement, rather than living in constant frustration at not having done better.

In my thirties I ran and swam and cycled regularly, but didn't fully enjoy the level of fitness I'd got to, because I was always agitated that I was still only half the speed of people who were really fit.

When I came off stage after an enjoyable show, I was often frustrated it hadn't gone better.

Whenever I played the piano in my clunky way, I felt mildly irritated that I couldn't play like professional jazz musicians, and so on.

Now I feel naturally joyful at any achievement, whether it's a scuffed goal in a game of five-a-side football or a session at the gym in which I repeatedly adjusted the machines so I was lifting 30 per cent of the weight of the growling man who'd been on them before me.

Now it seems tragic to be unable to enjoy achievements, except as a step towards a future situation that you *will* enjoy – 'I'm going to the gym because I'll be happy when I'm truly fit' or 'I'm working sixteen hours a day at something I dislike because I'll earn the money that will make me content.'

In the same way, campaigning for a cause or a charity isn't only a quest for an idyllic world; the striving for a different future transforms the present.

The battles to overthrow slavery or apartheid weren't only successful when they achieved their aims; they improved the lives of the victims of those situations during the conflict.

I think I have a greater capacity now to enjoy the process as well as the end result. In any case, a perfect outcome is an unattainable rainbow. The most revered classical pianists still have piano lessons. Usain Bolt, the week after he broke the 100-metres record, will have trained to become even faster. Beethoven wrote, shortly before he died, 'I feel I have scarcely written a note.' If you're unable to be satisfied at the point you've arrived at, you never will be satisfied.

I'm more likely now to sense the glory in any moment. Of course it makes sense for someone to start learning Italian in their eighties or take up the violin when they have a year to live. It doesn't matter that they'll never be perfect; they'll be better than they were before, and even if they're not, if they take pleasure from making an awful noise, that process should be celebrated.

*

It took me several months to realise that after my cancer treatment, I no longer felt in a rush. This seemed to make little sense. I'd become more aware of how time was limited, so I should have been in even more of a hurry.

Instead I feel the opposite: an acceptance that in a finite amount of time left alive, there is a finite amount that is possible to do, to experience.

I sometimes consider the alternate scenario to the one I'm in, the other world where Dr Oikonomou said, 'I'm afraid the scan has showed the cancer has spread into the lungs. There are still treatments we can try to slow down the process and you may still have two years but no more than that.'

In those circumstances, would I be revving my car at traffic lights, yelling at the person in front to 'hurry up, for fuck's sake, I've only got a year and five months to live so I don't want to waste any of it stuck behind you because you don't surge forward on amber'?

Few terminally ill people behave like this. Instead they seem to react to a lack of remaining time by rushing less, more likely to absorb each moment and take something from each situation, rather than see chunks of their life as worthless except as a means of getting them to the next moment that will possibly be worth living.

But strangely, none of this feels morbid. Having a peek at the possibility of imminent death may be the luckiest of experiences, as there's a joyfulness about accepting your demise.

It's too simplistic to suggest you learn to enjoy each day. You will still have days when you feel sad or wistful or useless, or exhausted for a reason you can't explain, or irritated by someone who walks slightly slower than you on a thin pavement and you can't get past the bastard. You'll still fume at websites covered in shite about the history of the company without telling you their address, or a packet of cheese that comes in three films of impregnable packaging. But now I seem to partly enjoy those experiences as an inevitable part of life that should be appreciated.

Making the most of every day doesn't mean taking up the oboe and learning to fly a helicopter; it can mean lying on the settee watching old episodes of *The Simpsons*.

The playwright Dennis Potter gave an interview when he was a few months from dying of cancer, in which he famously talked about a bush that he'd always enjoyed seeing, but now he was nearing his end, he said, the bush had the 'whitest frothiest blossomest blossom'.

I have had nothing approaching the stark consultation with death that he had, but now I think I understand better than before what he meant. I always liked the view out west from my bedroom. Now I love it.

I always enjoyed making my show about the towns. The series I made as I was recovering from the cancer treatment I absolutely loved. I have chosen to spend a chunk of my limited time doing this, and had Dr Oikonomou told me different news, I'd be doing something much less joyful than wandering around Stoke. I wasn't thinking any of this consciously, but it must have percolated in the back of my mind to make my days in Margate and East Grinstead more enjoyable, more blossomy.

A similar process took place with my closest relationships. I was already aware that I loved my son, daughter and granddaughter, but now if I'm reading *Spot the Dog* again to the three-year-old, I find myself thinking the actual words *This is AMAZING.**

Conversely, it created an urgent lack of interest in my biological family. I'd received two messages over the previous five years from my natural father, each in reply to a message I'd sent to him giving a few details of my life. Each of his emails was gentle and sympathetic, but the greatest

* I'm reminded of those people who said, 'I enjoyed the Covid lockdown because I got to know my kids.' Whenever I heard someone say that I thought, *It took a global pandemic to get you to know your own fucking kids? After six weeks of lockdown, did you find out you had one of each? 'Before that I thought they were both boys'?*

space was given to imploring me to no longer make our connection public, as he felt this could disrupt his current family, who he hadn't mentioned me to.

After my post-treatment scan, I wrote to tell him he was, biologically at least, a great-grandfather and that for the last nine months I'd been a cancer patient. He replied with a genial 'sorry about that' tone, adding that he'd once had similar treatment himself. But the bulk of his reply was another plea to not mention him in any public forum.

It might seem an unusual response to a blood relative telling you they're being treated for cancer, to take the opportunity to plead with them not to mention to anyone you're their relative.

Of all the unlikely and possibly inappropriate replies, it probably comes just behind 'sorry you've got cancer but can you lend me a hedge-trimmer', or 'if you've lost weight from the cancer, can you pop round and squeeze behind my freezer to find an earring I dropped there?'

With no sense of disappointment, I decided not to reply. There were so many people who had contacted me to express affection, jollity and spirit, who I would never get the time to converse properly with, what with time being finite because of the certainty of death, so why would I waste any more of my life on someone whose main concern regarding me was that I never mentioned he was anything to do with me?

My son had been a model carer throughout the ordeal. He hovered the optimum distance from me, watching like a lifeguard at an American beach, unnoticed until he could spot a problem he could help with, such as popping to the shop for tissues to wipe up the sick.

Among his accomplishments was to buy a suspicious device before I started the treatment, which allowed us to watch any sporting event live on TV, so I could take my mind off the mucus by watching Crystal Palace lose miserably.

Each day he told me about shows he'd taken part in, events at his jiujitsu gym, incidents that reminded me of an outside world that bounced defiantly on, regardless of my mucus. And he came with me to the critical appointments where we'd sit in waiting rooms, as he recounted with glee a disastrous gig his mate had suffered, with a cruelty that showed his compassion, as we sat in waiting rooms and I filled in forms to consent to have holes pierced in me.

Maybe his finest achievement was to never clasp my hand and tell me softly that everyone was thinking of me and 'this has made me realise what truly matters' – that would have made me doubt everything I'd ever done as a parent.

He wrote an hour-long show in which the cancer played a major part, which was acclaimed at the Edinburgh Festival with a series of exultant reviews.

Of course, most of us love our family members with an instinctive guttural passion, but we inevitably put that to one side. It's in the bank, it's guaranteed, so we can neglect the people close to us for a while as we strive for other, less certain goals. But if we're told we may be dying, we'll immediately think of the people closest to us and realise we'd assumed our time with them would go on for ever.

Or maybe there are people who would be told by a consultant, 'I'm afraid you only have six months,' and they would shout, 'Oh shit, now I'll NEVER beat Dave from accounts at golf.'

Little of this altered perspective on time is conscious. It creeps up on you. I found myself spending a day on the beach with my daughter and granddaughter that once would have been a day I had to write an article in response to an urgent email. Now I think the more urgent the email, the less urgent it really could be. If all the emails headed 'URGENT' in a whole day were ignored, would anyone notice?* With all these senses of urgency, the motivation wasn't that time was limited because I'd had cancer, it was that time is limited because it's ALWAYS FUCKING LIMITED. Awareness of the limited nature of time ironically made me in less of a daily rush. My co-comic-canceree Rhod Gilbert told me he felt so transformed by his experience, that however strange it sounds, he was glad of it. He also said he found that common among people who had recovered. For me, cancer seems an extreme way to sort out your priorities but I understand the logic. And maybe it is possible to act with this attitude before you get cancer. At Phil Jerrod's memorial, there were many laments for the tragedy of his death, but also a sense of celebration at this soul who had pulsated such warmth and humble eccentricity. Because in his mid-thirties he gave up a steady career working in a

* The answer is obviously 'yes', if they came from a nuclear power plant or a tsunami warning system or the lion enclosure of a zoo.

publishing office to pursue a calling in stand-up comedy. He was taken on by an agency and spent the next few years touring the country with his wonderfully structured disorder. And as the speeches were made, I was so glad that he'd taken the reckless decision at 35 to give up a steady career and instead pursue this notoriously unstable life. He could have delayed it, until the time was right, when the mortgage was more settled and the economic climate more favourable. He would still have got cancer, but his memorial would have been a series of people saying he was the funniest person who ever worked in the office and should have been on stage. I'm so glad he acted as if time was limited, before he found out so starkly that it was.

Eighteen

Love Letters

After my scans revealed I was still alive, I spoke to Jeremy Hardy's wife, Katy, who was typically sincerely inquiringly congratulatory.

She told me she had some notes that Jeremy had written in the months after his diagnosis and asked if I'd like to read them. So I cleared a morning and began to gaze at these words, having to pause every couple of minutes as I wasn't sure which emotion was catapulting me into an anaesthetised stupor, during which a surgeon could have operated on my liver and I wouldn't have felt a thing.

The most obvious reason why it was so disconcerting is that his descriptions were horribly familiar. He had a PET scan in the lorry outside the main building in St George's Hospital, exactly where I had mine. He describes the injection of blue dye and the warning not to be near pregnant women for four hours afterwards as he was a little bit radioactive.

In one meeting an oncologist said the MRI scan on his shoulder showed activity that was 'very suspicious', exactly the words of the doctor who took my biopsy.

A dietician ordered him boxes of the Fortisip drinks that I would become so intimate with. If we'd thought about it, I could have taken the ones he didn't use and kept them until I needed them myself.

The dietician suggested he added butter to everything to stop losing weight, just as one of them did to me four years later.

There's the same reading of faces, the waiting outside rooms for vital results. He wrote about one meeting, after he'd started chemotherapy that was targeting the cancer on his oesophagus. He had an endoscopy that he thought would be routine, but 'the endoscopist stopped briefly and said "I have some results" in a way that wasn't promising. Then he came back, ashen-faced, to tell me the cancer had metastasised to my bones.'

This was when he was told his probable prognosis was between eighteen months and two years, which began the two-week period when I couldn't reach him, when presumably he couldn't face telling people.

Reading this seemed doubly profound. On the one hand, because of my own experience, I now understood the details of what Jeremy went through, up until receiving the news that he probably wouldn't survive; the thought processes, the bit of the stomach that tightens, the numb walk back to the car, the sharp jolts of guilt as you imagine telling your family.

I could picture him, in one of those functional chairs, searching for the question that might elicit some hope as a nurse stood helplessly holding a clipboard. I could feel him struggling to hear the details of the notes and the appointments that would be made as he turned this news around in his head.

But also, more selfishly, I understood, because of his experience, how few steps away I was from hearing similar news. I had all those discussions, past the acknowledgement of cancer and the revelation via a mistake or two that it was secondary cancer.

I'm glad I didn't understand at the time the significance of the word 'metastasise'.

When I was told my cancer had metastasised I thought it sounded quite cheerful.

Jeremy was always far more etymologically proficient than I was so he'd have known what it meant, that it had spread.

It was only when I was told it hadn't metastasised into my lungs that I knew I was on a probable road to safety, and though I knew this was a big moment, I had no idea at the time it was *that* big.

I was still one piece of bad news away from a vastly shortened life, whereas Jeremy never got his first win of the season.

He finishes this section by saying he was still clinging to hope. He wrote, 'I'm still hoping to receive a phone call from my hearty oncologist saying, "I'm sorry we've put you through a lot of rather gruelling, and, it turns out, superfluous, chemo; but it seems the lab mixed up your biopsy with someone else's and you don't have Stage 4 Oesophageal Cancer at all. So, good news! And now I have to make a rather awkward call to a Mrs Geraldine Harty."'

As I read it, I wasn't sure whether to feel grateful my situation was different or sickeningly sad that his wasn't.

*

Among the contradictions that Jeremy seemed to experience was his reluctance, as the humble soul he was, to discuss his situation, along with the impulse as a writer and comic to tell everyone.

For example, he wrote, 'I detest all the language about "beating the Big C". For one thing, grow up and call it by its name, and for another, I can't beat it. I'm the patient.

'It lives in my body but I don't control it. I'm not growing it on purpose. I'm not a fucking allotment. Stop talking about fighting cancer, as though I've got to train somehow, as though for a marathon. And if I die, don't tell me I've lost my battle with it, as though I'm a failure as well as a corpse.'

This is obviously fairly angry, but I don't think it means the cancer made him angry.

Instead he carried what made him angry anyway into his new situation. Pomposity made him angry when it was displayed by an advertising executive or a middle-aged couple that's moved to the countryside and now 'can't understand why anyone would live in the city'.

I sensed an honour in his anger, because I was more selfish and turned away from what might fuel those thoughts. If anything required my anger, it would have to wait until I was cured. I didn't have the capacity to be angry about the many things that it's right to be angry about, but Jeremy appears to have carried on being angry, almost out of a sense of duty.

He was furious with people who offered him holistic 'alternative' cures, saying he was 'sick of people telling me there's a plant that was given to someone who was beheaded by ISIS and now they're fine'.

And he wrote, 'I got into text spats with friends who are annoying me by constantly proffering unasked-for advice. I had to make it clear that all these "I know someone who was dead and now they're alive again – technically it was a zombie film I saw, but I stand by my point" people are just depressing me.

'Also don't say, "I want to give you a big hug", unless your hugs have been peer-reviewed and proven to be of some benefit.'

And on being told he had probably between a year and 18 months, he wrote that his thoughts were, 'Never mind me. I must not fail the people I love, love more now than I have ever loved them, and to whom I owe so much. I have to stick around for them. Even if it gets to the point that my life seems awful to me, if I can still be something for them, and if they would still rather have me than not, I have to try. I have to fight this bloody cancer and be the hero I've never been. And when I lose the fight, at least I'll take this bloody cancer with me, so what will it have won?'

He'd seemed so magnificently defiant and yet here he was with all the fears and regrets, crushing disappointments and sickening acceptance that any one of us would have.

It was so hard to read; each paragraph had an impact slightly deeper than the last as I felt those thoughts tipping out of him, some of them contradictory, such as his proclamation that he'll fight the cancer after he had fumed that it was not a battle.

And yet they all made perfect sense, as a beautiful scream that he wanted to live but knew he wouldn't and was trying to make sense of what he knew couldn't be made sense of. And mostly he wanted to do that for people other than himself.

Again it all seemed so much closer than it had before I knew the smell and the sweat of those corridors, and I felt his words as I hadn't or couldn't have at the time he wrote them.

When his friend the comic Jack Dee wheeled him into a meeting with the oncologist, he wrote, 'Jack came up to the unit and I introduced him to Lydia, saying, "This is Jack, he's on work experience – for when he gets cancer."' By the time I'd finished reading, I felt like the child in the film *AI* who gets to meet his digitally resurrected dead mother for just one day before she disappears again for ever.

Nineteen

Last Christmas

A few weeks after my 'all-clear' call, I was asked to be the guest on *Desert Island Discs*, the iconic radio show first broadcast in 1942, in which 'castaways' must choose the eight records they would take with them if they were to be stranded alone on a desert island.

This seemed like a massive honour, or responsibility. My daughter screamed with delight when I told her, then started proposing songs. Other friends did the same, and Shappi suggested the programme's producers didn't know about my latest scan result and thought, *We'd better get him quick in case we don't get another chance.*

She asked how I would choose my discs, adding, 'If it was me, the first one I'd choose would be "Valentine" by Willie Nelson,' and I shook a bit.

I asked her to meet me, adding, 'You can't say no as I've had cancer.'

We went to see a show and began, during the interval, to explain the times we'd had, the psychotherapy course that had been central to her life and the radiotherapy course that had been central to mine.

She had realised, she told me, that she had become aware, explosively, that she had to be single.

Infuriatingly it was about then that the second half of the show began.

Afterwards she told me she was a little shocked at how much weight I'd lost, and how I couldn't hear properly and ate so slowly and I rapidly saw the previous year from her perspective, that someone she loved was undergoing this trial and she couldn't communicate with them; it wasn't dissimilar from having a loved one in intensive care during Covid.

She couldn't sleep, she said, and sometimes wondered whether she should have just burst into the hospital ward unannounced, like a superhero.

And I felt a strange sense of guilt in that I couldn't have done anything differently but still felt terrible for having done it. I couldn't risk facing the dual drama of disease and a tempestuous love affair. Even the Stoics would have said, 'We're not THAT fucking stoic.'

And I wondered how we had got into such a pickle that at every point one of us had been unable to communicate with the other – sometimes her, sometimes me, sometimes both. It happens because until we're forced to confront the reality of mortality, we think there's always boundless time. So we have the luxury of acting as if we can ignore someone to make a point or dismiss our feelings while we reorganise ourselves or be driven by a sense of rejection or a need to blame, or because we want to get someone back for hurting us, and there's no better cure for that than being made brutally aware there's no guarantee you will ever see this person alive for an extra minute.

We agreed to go away for the weekend, just as friends, and I was immediately amazed by her expansive enthusiasm for something, anything, everything and the exact words didn't matter; what mattered was the exuberance and the mischief.

Immediately it felt as if we were a couple as she smiled at me directly, the way you do with a tiny handful of people in your life, and I picked flecks of cotton off her shirt.

By now 20 years of affection culminating in a cancer-addled year of torment had matured into a deep sense of belonging; we held hands on a promenade and both promised to sort it this time.

This isn't to ignore the old tensions but to accept them, as you have to accept the cannula and the mask, and find the best way of getting through them.

I'm not sure this would have been possible without the cancer, so thank you, cancer, for helping to sort us out.

*

After I was given the results of the scan, that the treatment had burned away the tumour, all I had to do was be careful not to catch cancer again and I'd be fine.

I wasn't sure if this meant I was officially cured or if I was in the state that I'd heard mentioned in other cases: 'remission'.

I'd never understood what 'in remission' meant. It sounded like the cancer had taken some time off, maybe to do a course at college or to recover by the seaside after having a nervous breakdown, following the stress of being irradiated every day for six weeks.

Maybe the three-monthly scans would be like an MOT for a car, so occasionally they would have to renew a few cells or refit a lymph node to get me through, the equivalent of changing a tyre.

During the days of my mucus eruptions I'd had the notion (it must have been in one of those recesses as I was admiring the view of Twickenham in the distance) that if

I came through this I would have a party in the summer, to replace the Christmas I lost.

So after the scan result, I booked a room at a cafe in Crystal Palace Park for 19 July and sent out invites that my daughter designed.

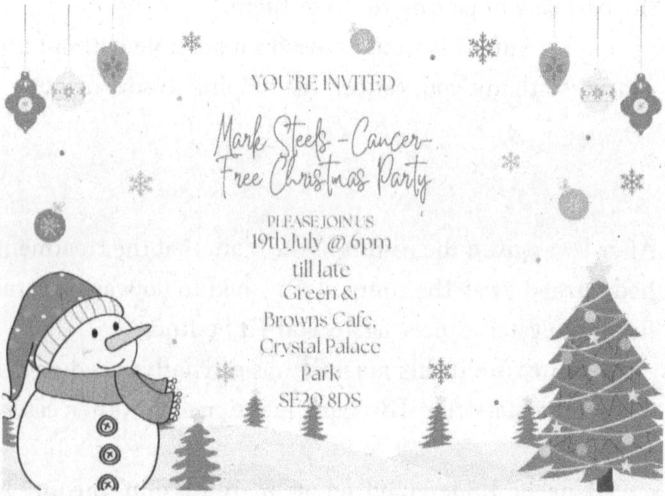
YOU'RE INVITED
Mark Steels – Cancer-Free Christmas Party
PLEASE JOIN US
19th July @ 6pm
till late
Green &
Browns Cafe,
Crystal Palace
Park
SE20 8DS

I ordered a tree from Argos and picked it up at the store in Streatham, from a young woman who said with such confusion she was almost angry, 'You know, like, it's summer and that, like, why are you buying a Christmas tree?'

With the people who had been so critical to getting through all this, we had turkey and stuffing and Brussels sprouts and pulled crackers and played Christmas songs in the stifling July heat.

Jules and his wife Jo came, the first time I'd seen them since his message about his unwelcome scan results, and they were obscenely cheerful and optimistic and delighted with my progress. Could I have been that positive in those circumstances?

Could I have attended a 'cancer-free' party of someone with whom I was treated for cancer when I wasn't cancer-free?

'Whatever the outcome of all this,' he told me and a group of friends, 'I want to leave something positive for my kids out of it.'

That impressed me enormously. It was one thing to say that a few months ago, back then it was in theory, but to say it in this situation was far cooler.

Jules mentioned he was having a hormone treatment that was reducing his testosterone levels. 'I suppose the next stage is I'll be changing my pronouns,' he said. That's a fine joke from anyone but somehow it's spectacular when said by a general in the British Army.

The couple told us of some of the awkward conversations they've been forced into. 'Our eldest son, who's 16, asked, "If Dad dies, will we get a new dad one day?"'

Among the avalanche of uncertainties cascading through this lad's mind, this must have forced its way forward and popped out in words.

'So we thought about it,' said Jules and Jo, in that way that some couples seem to collaborate with such efficient affection they appear to think as a single organism, 'and I didn't want any possible unease in the future, so I said, "None of you should live lives defined by my death." Then I said, "Mind you, that doesn't mean your mum can go on Tinder five minutes after the funeral."'

At least two people listening tried to hide a tear as they laughed at this contender for joke of the year.

*

I couldn't have imagined this party six months earlier. I had the idea for it but was literally unable to picture it. It felt it would have been counterproductive to dream about it; it seemed too distant from where I was, as fanciful as someone imagining winning an Olympic marathon as they're fighting an addiction to Yorkie bars and have just bought their first pair of trainers.

There seemed to be no connection between the two worlds, of then and now. Was I the same person? I was glad it took me an hour to eat a turkey leg as that was the only evidence it was me that had been through the events of the previous winter.

A few days before the Christmas party, I'd had another MRI scan, the second of my three-monthly sessions. Even more mundane than the first, it was conducted with a matter-of-fact sigh and I'm sure the nurse puffed out her cheeks as I climbed out of the machine, as if she worked in a car wash and had just wiped her 35th dashboard of the day.

This time I couldn't put the people I knew through the same drama as I had while waiting for the results of the first scan. I wasn't sure of the rules about how much anxiety it's permissible to exude when you're waiting for the second one. What must it be like when it gets to the eleventh scan? By then it's three years and nine months since the treatment ended, so you probably pop into it on the way to Morrisons. But any one of these scans could, in theory, show that the cancer had returned and more treatment would be needed, that you'd be an active cancer patient again.

This time I asked Shappi to be around on the morning that I got the results. Perhaps I would come to share this job around so after four years I'd be asking the nice lady from the dry cleaner's.

The phone rang, the same dry but sensitive soul told me what the scan had revealed, saying the enlarged lymph node that was their only concern had shrunk and no other problems were apparent. Then he said he would order a PET scan, the 'Rolls-Royce of scans' that I'd first come into contact with about a year earlier.

This would examine not just the area that the cancer was in but my whole body and if this was clear as well, I would be off the books and require no more scans at all. This seemed wonderful: I was *so* un-cancerous I didn't even need regular checking.

The next afternoon I was in Paris, watching England play South Africa in an Olympic women's hockey match. As my phone rang I recognised it was a hospital number and a secretary gave me a date to have this scan.

I wasn't expecting that. This was *too* quick and efficient. Why were they in such a rush? They seemed so eager I wondered if they were planning to bring the scan to the hockey.

And so my mind twisted into the spiral of uncertainty and speculation I recognised from a year before. A PET scan? They didn't give those away cheaply, just in case.

What did they suspect? Had they got an inkling my neck was free of cancer but it had relocated, back to its primary home like someone in middle age who leaves the excitement of London, where they've lived since they were 19, to move back to Wiltshire, where they were brought up?

By the time England equalised with a wonderful looping thwack, I was able to replace these thoughts with, *I expect they're just being thorough.* Then the fretting would find a way through – *there was no suggestion of a PET scan before* – before my thoughts settled into a clinical *there's no point in guessing*, and I'd try to leave them there.

The PET scan took a morning, and by now I was used to the routine in which you get out of this magical machine in which your whole lifeline has been placed, and a dispassionate, slightly hurried radiographer points to the locker and reminds you not to forget your keys.

Then you wait. The app gave me a meeting in four weeks' time to discuss the results. How should I order my thoughts? Do I opt for *Of course it's fine, this is just a routine check, they told me, they'd bring me in much quicker if anything was wrong?*

Or do I go for *Whatever the results show, they won't be any different if I spend the next four weeks in a flap?*

To add to the drama, the appointment was on the same day that I was trying out, for the first time, my new show about my year as a cancer patient.

Normally I would arrive at the theatre around 4pm, which was the time the meeting with the consultant was due to begin.

If it started late, I might be the first person in history to be in a meeting fretting about cancer results at the same time as panicking about getting away to do a show in Reading.

Most of the four weeks behaved themselves. I spent a delightful week in the Isle of Wight with Shappi, I went to a couple of festivals, I wrote and ate and ran and performed and the scan results were barely noticeable, playing in an upstairs room, looking after themselves and needing only to be checked in on once every few days.

Throughout this time, my son, my daughter and Shappi insisted whenever I mentioned my concerns that I was worrying needlessly, I was clearly healthy, and it was obviously just a routine check-up.

But the day before the results meeting, the jitters came crashing in, bullying their way through all the calm and soft thoughts that were playing so nicely. Of all the states to accept, uncertainty seems to be the toughest. Now I swung wildly from *of course it's alright* to *it's probably serious* and back again.

Apart from anything else, what a fraud that Christmas party would turn out to be if I discovered the cancer had spread after all. I'd feel like someone who has a huge wedding, bringing people from hundreds of miles, then files for divorce six weeks later.

*

As I sat in the waiting room at the Macmillan Cancer Centre, behind me was a woman who didn't stop talking angrily about her mum for 20 minutes, to her friend who kept saying 'hmmm'. A doctor wearing a name tag bought a coffee. By the next afternoon he'd probably forgotten everything about this moment that would be crystallised in my mind for ever.

I waited for my name to appear on a screen, silently. I could sense the sweat under the armpits. At 30 minutes after the meeting should have started, I added the supplementary panic that I would be late for my show. Would it be healthy to panic about that instead?

As I waited to be called in, a dietician asked me to chat to her about how my eating was going. That was an efficient use of time but displayed an appalling lack of a sense of drama. All the tension was punctured as I chatted to her about how I was now able to eat a sausage.

We discussed the speed at which I could swallow a pint of beer and I tried not to be distracted by my impending meeting about whether I was full of deadly disease. If that meeting went badly, discussing my ability to swallow beer would be like a mechanic telling you the car would have to be crushed for scrap metal, but first they'd like to ask if I had any trouble with the windscreen wipers.

Then I was ushered in to see an imperious doctor who also asked about sausages and beer and biscuits and custard and said my voice sounded deeper and then mentioned, almost threw away, that the PET scan had revealed no sign of the primary cancer, that had probably disappeared for ever, then asked where the show was that night.

She was a fantastic doctor, but again, where was her sense of theatre?

You can't toss away the critical conclusion of the whole scene like that. Agatha Christie stories don't end with the detective saying, 'I hope you've all been eating well as I know it can be stressful being a murder suspect. Also, I worked out the gardener did it – would anyone fancy a biscuit?'

I had a swollen lymph node that was stubbornly resisting the treatment, but was only 8 millimetres bigger than normal; I would need to have that scanned again, but it wasn't much of a worry.

Then we talked about my vocal cords and I didn't have the heart to tell this glorious soul that inside I was puffing like a zebra that's just escaped a lion so I didn't really give a fuck about the nuances of my vocal cords.

And she put a camera up a nostril and down my throat, maybe for old time's sake, and it was searingly uncomfortable and a tear of discomfort glistened in each eye and I tried to recall that, for several months, this sort of thing had been as normal as washing my hands.

As the camera cable wiggled where my tonsils once were, I noticed it was 5.15, around the time I would normally be backstage at the theatre.

A few moments later they all wished me luck for the show, I left the hospital and saw that my son, my daughter and Shappi had all called. And as I told them my results, all three of them replied by exhaling a huge 'Oh, thank god' and told me they'd been more worried about these results than anything to do with my health for the last six months.

Twenty

Let's Stick Together

Sometimes, through the steam I was inhaling, my head face down in a bowl on a table, past the mist in my field of vision, was the array of boxes, bottles, tubes and flasks arranged on my kitchen table. They were an artistic blend of colours and in the haze resembled an impressionist painting that might be called *The Cure*. And I would wonder how much all this cost.

The idea that health care is free is so rooted into the psyche of Britain that we have to make an effort to acknowledge it. It's routine to complain about an awful doctor or an incompetent receptionist without recalling that this service is free, like almost nothing else.

You can't imagine complaining that 'the garage gave me a new car for free today. They kept me waiting twenty minutes and the radio doesn't work properly, they're a bloody disgrace.'

This is why one of the most moving pieces of literature in the English language is the leaflet distributed by the government in 1948, explaining how the National Health Service would work.

It had to state boldly: 'When you have chosen your doctor, he will not charge you fees.'

This was repeated in every section because so many people couldn't grasp the concept at all. My grandmother told of how some people couldn't understand the idea at the time, so when they received a pair of glasses from the NHS they would ask many times who they had to pay.

The idea that it was 'no one' was so absurd they couldn't grasp it. They were convinced they were simply confused about the new system. They would listen again to the explanation of National Insurance and central funds and patients not having to pay, then say again, 'But WHO do I pay?'

Because once a routine is firmly established in people's lives, it takes a massive rift to change it.

For example, around the seventeenth century in most of Britain there was a practice known as 'Saint Monday'. Many people's working week flowed with the rhythm of the market, which took place on a Saturday. So as long as all the clothing or whatever they were selling was ready by then, it didn't matter at what point of the week the work had been done. This meant they followed the beats of anyone with a deadline: getting behind until a mad scurry at the last minute. On Mondays most people didn't work at all, declaring it a holiday for Saint Monday, a little joke in honour of procrastination.

In the nineteenth century the factory system was established, with a new working practice that demanded you worked every hour you were employed to work for your employer. But in many towns the workforce carried on staying at home every Monday. The factory owners would refuse to pay them but it made no difference. It was rooted in the minds of millions of people that they didn't work on Mondays. You didn't, you just didn't. You might as well announce that from now on we must all walk backwards.

In some areas, such as the West Midlands, this went on until the second half of the nineteenth century, to the exasperation of the employers.

Similarly, we paid for health care, just like we paid for food or beer. We either paid for it when we used it or we paid into an insurance scheme.

Then all of a sudden we didn't, and it took a massive programme of explaining to establish this.

Now we accept as natural that childbirth or vaccinations or cancer treatment are without a charge, as much as it was once natural to pay for it.

For almost anyone born before the 1970s, it was beyond debate that the welfare state was a huge advance in society. Our parents and grandparents shared memories of friends and neighbours suffering and dying from lack of access to basic medicine. Or they would talk of having to pawn their clothing to buy a set of glasses. Anyone suggesting we should go back to the old system would sound as daft as someone saying we should reintroduce the plague, or scrap toilets and go back to chucking piss out of the window.

I used to do a bit in my show about the people who are infuriated by paying for services as a society, because we should be responsible only for our own individual needs. So they'd ask, 'Why should I pay for a health service when I'M NOT ILL, and why am I paying for a fire brigade when I'M NOT ON FIRE, and look at the money we waste on guide dogs! I can't climb trees but nobody buys me a gibbon.'

Even if you did measure your life in such an obsessive way, and never once needed the health service, you've still gained from it because you have never had to worry how you'd manage if you suddenly *were* in need of major treatment. The health service doesn't just remove the actual cost of health care from the individual, it removes the fear of it before it happens.

But now it had happened to me and I was peering through the wispy steam at boxes that clogged up 30 per cent of the kitchen, thinking, *How much have they had to pay for all that muck?*

A few times the doctor at the hospital gave me prescriptions, providing me with medicines I didn't think I'd need, so I would think, *Please don't, that will be a waste of money*, like a child imploring their grandma not to buy them an Airfix kit they know they'll never make.

All these sentiments must be unknown in a society where health is primarily a business. It seems nonsensical when politicians in the US argue against state-funded healthcare, by claiming this would 'remove choice'.

I imagine Republican supporters shouting that if they have cancer, they would hate to be under the British system where they're treated automatically, rather than given the choice of selling all their belongings to pay for chemotherapy, or dying.

There was a sketch made for YouTube about how the wonderful drama *Breaking Bad* would go if it was set in Britain. (In the show, chemistry teacher Walter White is diagnosed with cancer, so to fund his treatment he makes and sells crystal meth, which sparks six extraordinary series of craziness and intrigue.)

In the British version the doctor says, 'I'm afraid you have lung cancer. This is the team that will be dealing with you.' – The End.

The NHS didn't appear naturally; it was formed against the opposition of similar forces to the ones that prevent socialised healthcare in the United States. It was fought for by the people who created a sense that after the Second World War, a new society must be created.

George Orwell wrote in 1944 of the overwhelming sentiment in Britain that it was the lower classes that had made it possible for the war to be won, so when the war was over, they would demand and create a redefined Britain, transformed from the one of mass unemployment and poverty that preceded the war.

The battalions of old Britain, those that protested a welfare state would benefit only the idle, or that a health service would destroy 'choice', had to be confronted.

And my face full of steam to deal with the eruptions of mucus following blasts of radiotherapy was thanks to those that won that confrontation.

*

It's impossible to calculate accurately the cost of anyone's treatment. You would have to take into account the expense of building the hospital, of maintenance, cleaning, insurance, energy bills, window cleaning, stationery, the wages for porters, cooks and drivers who delivered the machines you used and then decide what portion of this was down to your specific treatment.

We can say that my course of radiotherapy would cost £3,000 if it was carried out by a private clinic. And the chemo would cost the same. A PET scan would cost

£2,500 (I had two of those) and an MRI scan £250 (I had six of those).

I had a two-and-a-half-hour operation to remove the lump in my throat and my tonsils, and tonsil removals are charged at £2,550 (I presume that's for both - and I hope there's a special offer, such as three tonsils for the price of two).

The removal of tonsils was the minor part of my operation, so I expect the whole job would be charged at a much higher rate. Then there were the sessions with a wide array of medical staff, maybe 50 altogether, that would be charged at between £100 and £300 each.

There were 14 nights in the hospital and all the drugs displayed on my table.

And the boxes of syringeable liquid jollifying the kitchen. It would probably have cost somewhere between £50,000 and £100,000 in total.

For the private health companies, it's a disaster if the National Health Service is wonderfully efficient. Selling anything is tricky, but it must be more difficult if the product you're marketing can be obtained elsewhere, better than yours, and for free.

Maybe that's why an article in the *Daily Mail* about the difference between private and public cancer treatments mentioned that the private London Clinic boasts, 'Artisan hams and edible flowers are a feature of the meals that their patients could enjoy.'

If only I could have afforded it, I could have watched artisan hams and edible flowers get wheeled out on a trolley, so I could have pointed to the 'nil by mouth' card above my bed before the porter went 'oh yeah' and took them away again.

*

The University College Hospital building is at the north end of Tottenham Court Road in central London, a few hundred yards from the BT Tower.

It was founded in 1745 for the 'sick and lame of Soho'. During the most tumultuous days of the French Revolution, it dedicated two wards to the French clergy who were fleeing their country.

I expect there was an outcry of people complaining that 'we should look after our own sick and lame, not these people claiming to be sick and lame from some war or other' and telling us, 'You don't hear English no more round there, it's all bloody Latin up Soho these days.'

It's an area whose history hides behind the constant scurrying of modern life that rattles past its exhibits without a glance.

A million people a day must stride down Gower Street, possibly unaware that Charles Darwin lived in a flat above them.

The fully dressed skeleton of philosopher Jeremy Bentham, who taught that all thought and action must be judged by its consequences, is displayed in the Student Centre at University College London, near the ear and dentist wing of the hospital.

Karl Marx lived in nearby Dean Street and once had to flee the police, who pursued him for drunkenly throwing stones at a gaslight on the street where I meandered in an addled daze, due to morphine I'd been given for free by the state a few yards away, an act that Marx would probably have considered *too* communist.

In the hospital itself, George Orwell spent his last days dying of TB. And Agatha Christie took a job in the hospital pharmacy, maybe to learn about poisons to help with her murder stories.

I have a vague memory of visiting my granddad, who was dying of lung cancer in 1967, at the old site of the hospital on Fitzroy Street. My dad took me up the Post Office Tower (now BT Tower) as a treat before seeing Granddad for the last time, an act that has cemented the pair (Granddad and the Post Office Tower) as bound together in my mind.

Now, 57 years later, the new hospital building puffs out its glass chest as the dominant construction in the area, perched on the edge of the unfathomable dual carriageway, underpass and bewildering crossroads of Euston Road.

There are 14 wide storeys that must make developers wince, as each bed space could be a studio flat worth a million pounds.

Then there are two more floors underground that could so easily be a car park or a gym for the residents, instead of housing the radiotherapy department where absolutely anyone can saunter in, put on a mask and get their tumour irradiated.

A & E is directly in front of the main road, so patients, waiting for the dramatic moment when their name is called, can gaze at the lines of traffic, staying still like the most stubborn donkey as the Gower Street lights turn from red to green and back again, maybe wondering whether it's the people inside or outside the building who will be the first to make any progress.

*

A few yards away from the main building is the Macmillan Cancer Centre, a £110 million building opened in 2012, modern and glass with a vast open-plan reception area and a spiral staircase leading to the arty chemo room. And the whole building is dedicated to cancer, so you don't have to share it with patients of lesser diseases, which always cheapens the cancer day out.

The centre receives extra funding because much of its work is dedicated to research, and the hospital as a whole has its funding supplemented because it's a teaching hospital, a centre of medical training.

It's often suggested by governments that 'the problems within the health service can't simply be solved by throwing money at it'.

This is true of any problem. If you have a car that's broken down, you don't simply get it working again by throwing money at it. BUT IT FUCKING HELPS.

If you've only got five pounds, it's a lot more difficult to replace an engine than if you can afford to pay Max Verstappen's personal mechanic and tell him to put in as many new engines as he likes.

Some problems, such as nurses and junior doctors having less money in real terms than they did ten years ago, you can clearly solve by throwing money at them, because the problem they have is that not enough money has been thrown at them.

It's true that money wouldn't solve every problem. When I went to those meetings in which I was finding out my predicted fate, there was an unsettling disorder as soon as you arrived, as a puzzling gathering hovered around a counter before a flustered receptionist who lifted up and put down clipboards as she looked for notes she was sure she'd put here somewhere.

Then someone in the semi-queue would call out, 'Any news of Dr Sharma?' And the receptionist would slide further into that whirlpool of having to deal with five issues at once. I imagine it's like when you're attending to a five-year-old who's crying because they've lost their fluffy rabbit and trapped their fingers in a door while you're late for a train, then the nine-year-old cries, 'Dad! The internet's not working.'

I wouldn't have blamed the receptionist if she'd yelled, 'CAN'T YOU SEE I'M BUSY? DEAL WITH YOUR OWN BLOCKED OESOPHAGUS!' As I was there to discover whether my PET scan had revealed if my cancer had spread or not, I simply withdrew into my own world and tried to block out the chaotic orchestra around me.

From the time I was assigned to UCH I never had to meditate my way out of a cacophony like this again.

For example, every time I arrived for one of my 30 radiotherapy sessions, a receptionist said brightly, 'You're in booth D today, Mr Steel,' then tapped something on her laptop to register I'd arrived.

Maybe the receptionists there were trained more thoroughly to be welcoming to patients, or perhaps they did yoga and knew how to regulate their breathing to stay positive. But a huge factor in them remaining cheerful was that there were two of them. So if one was detained by an irritating laptop disorder or a patient who couldn't remember his address, the other one could greet everyone as normal.

The receptionist was more likely to stay cheerful because money had been thrown to make sure there were two of them.

*

On the day I had my ears tested before the treatment started, I noticed a line of paintings along the walls of the waiting room, some of them depicting crowds of people in London, others a blend of swirling purple lines, the sort of thing that makes me struggle not to say out loud, 'What the bloody hell is that?'

But all the paintings spoke to me in one way, which was that someone had taken the trouble to choose them and to hang them up. The walls could have been left bare, or covered in posters still warning about Covid or rabies. Or they could have been decorated with slightly skewwhiff paintings of dogs playing snooker and no one would complain.

But on these walls were paintings that someone had taken care over. The hospital takes so much care that they employ an art curator, who has worked with Grayson Perry and Peter Blake, artists so well known that I've heard of them.

You don't need much imagination to picture the fuming outrage. An art curator? In a bloody hospital? No wonder they're short of funds, they're supposed to be taking out your manky appendix, not curating poxy purple circles.

I looked at the poxy purple circles, trying to understand what they were for, wondering if I was simply meant to appreciate the vivid colours. I was still considering this when I was called in for my ear test, exactly on time, which was a shame as there were other paintings I was looking forward to peering at.

*

At Croydon hospital, where I began my cancer process, at the entrance is a gloomy Costa Coffee that must have been specially designed to emit extra gloom. At a chipped table you remove the cardboard remains of the last person to sit there and queue behind one other person for 15 minutes until someone returns to serve you, by which time you have to leave without a coffee as it's time for your appointment, which you arrive at feeling that you're already surrounded by a puff of despair.

I got lost on the way to my MRI scan. There was a pink line painted around the wall, which I was told to follow as it would lead to the imaging department. It jiggled along corridors, round alcoves, onto the floor, then stopped by a door that looked like a fire escape. I went outside, where I wondered if a wizard would give me a clue to get to the next stage.

I went across a path between some long grass, into

another part of the building where the pink line started again. Sometimes it joined with a yellow or green line before sharply changing direction, as if it was playing a children's game of 'tag' and was determined not to be caught.

I followed it round several more corners, past a chemist, a chapel and a toilet, where it suddenly stopped. I met another man looking equally puzzled and we joined together to search for the missing pink line. Maybe we would have to take a 'leap of faith' like Indiana Jones and we'd land right by the scanning machine.

Eventually someone in a white coat asked if we were looking for the imaging department. We said that we were, and they directed us, saying the pink line was painted over a couple of years ago and they haven't got round to putting it back.

Maybe, if they can't find the time or paint to redraw the pink line that's gone missing, they should just call it *Broken Pink Line* and say it's a work of art they've curated.

*

In the week before my radiotherapy and chemo began, I was called by someone from UCH who ran through the possible claims I could make if my treatment left me unable to cope financially. She would help me fill in the forms, she said, because they can be highly confusing.

She was so determined to help that I wanted to ask if she could help filling in other forms, such as the one to renew my car insurance and one claiming compensation for a train that got in late from Sheffield.

I couldn't make any claim but she still helped enormously, because she became part of an assurance that every angle of my illness was being considered. They could offer all this ingenious technology to blast away my tumour, but if I panicked after three weeks because I was hopelessly in debt and stopped coming to the treatment, the whole process would be pointless. Of course that wouldn't happen. But one month earlier, as I was driving to Tooting for my first PET scan, I was half-listening to the Radio 5 Live morning phone-in show with Nicky Campbell. The topic of the day was that a survey had revealed a record number of days off sick had been taken by the country's workforce over the previous year.

So of course there was a call from an angry man, furious because 'I can't have a day off as I'm self-employed, not like these teachers and people these days, my dad never had a day off in his life, in the old days you didn't skive off with a sniffle' and so on, that made me want to call in and reply that I was a lumberjack and once sawed myself clean in half up a tree with a chainsaw, but the bottom half still went in every day and chopped down an entire forest in the Yukon.

Then a cab driver came on to say he'd been diagnosed with cancer and was put on a course of radiotherapy, similar to the one I was destined for. He'd hoped the treatment would take place early in the morning so he could get it done each day before work. This went well for the first two weeks, but then the times of his treatment were changed to later in the day so he stopped going as he couldn't afford to take time off.

I don't often yell into the air at people on phone-in shows, but I made an exception for him. I howled into the void, 'NOOOO, no no no, have you got a son, a daughter, a mum, a neighbour who can feed you for two months? The treatment isn't optional; if you don't have it, you'll die, you idiot!'

The rent was his biggest problem, he said. And so it was that thousands of years of biological advances, from Aristotle's theories of a body driven by humours, through the analysis of corpses during the Renaissance and the understanding that the heart drove blood around the body, on to the great discoveries of penicillin, X-rays, and ultimately the technology of micro-surgery and PET scans, were all rendered worthless because when the treatment was offered the poor sod couldn't afford the time off to go and take it.

The wonders of science and the glory of the NHS couldn't compete with the demands of the cab driver's landlord.

The ingenuity of any medical team has to battle against the world outside as well as the disease they're confronting in the patient's body.

I was relatively privileged, certainly compared to the sick cab driver. But in the days before my operation I had to calculate the impact of earning no money for at least six months and arrange with the bank to take that time off paying the mortgage.

Along with all the other issues that invaded my mind at this time, I pledged to do the sensible thing and ignore all financial problems completely until all this was finished.

I think I figured that if I got through this alright I'd be so relieved, I wouldn't be bothered that I was six months behind with every bill imaginable. Maybe a bit of me thought that whatever we think about banks and energy companies, surely they let you have everything for free if you've had cancer.

But I could find ways of ignoring all this, whereas the cab driver probably couldn't ignore an angry landlord, maybe stood at his door with an Alsatian.

*

The external problems that seem so important until you get cancer are still important once you've got cancer. It won't help your ability to deal with cancer if you're evicted from your flat.

Your individual circumstances and environment will continue to be real and they will have a huge bearing on how you cope with the ordeal chucked at you.

As is so often the case, all these thoughts seemed particularly poignant as I learned more about East Grinstead.

In the days approaching my scan results, I was reading about the small West Sussex town for my radio show, and came across the practices of Archibald McIndoe, a plastic surgeon from New Zealand who came to Britain in the 1930s.

Plastic surgery was in its infancy; most people who suffered severe burns died fairly quickly, so there was little point in attending to their appearance. But an improved understanding of the effect of burns led to new techniques that could keep patients alive.

At this point Archibald was sent to East Grinstead hospital, a centre of plastic surgery. The town had been chosen as a site for this branch of medicine by the plastic surgeon Sir Harold Gillies, because it was halfway between his house in London and his golf club in Rye.

But it turned out to be a fine choice. In 1940 the air battles of the Second World War sent hundreds of burned airmen to the hospital, where Archibald was in charge of rebuilding their burned and disfigured bodies and faces. This is when he implemented his radical approach.

He insisted that for the patients to recover, their mental state had to be as positive as possible. The airmen had been through the most excruciating trauma, and were now horribly disfigured. Even if they survived and the plastic surgery was successful, they would spend their lives permanently scarred. If they couldn't overcome the mental anguish attached to this, they wouldn't be capable of the physical ordeal of recovering, he said.

So he ordered that officers and lower ranks were treated together on the wards. He insisted there was a constant supply of beer and cigarettes in the ward. (I had no idea that the Polish man who lit up in the cancer ward was only following the example of Archibald McIndoe.)

He wanted his ward to feel as if it was a constant party, and the ward became known as 'The Guinea Pig Club'.

Every day, staff and patients would toast the club with glasses of sherry.

Among the accounts of patients was one from Harold Taubman, who said, 'I woke up on the first day at East Grinstead, the patient in the next bed said "have a cigar". A man in a wheelchair chased a nurse, shouting "taxi, taxi" and there was the lovely sound of the pouring of bottles of beer.'

In a statement that might not appear appropriate in a modern setting, Archibald wrote that 'all the nurses should be pretty'.

And he added, 'The matron must not mind when patients return from the nightclubs of London for breakfast.'

The most famous entertainers of the time, such as Tommy Trinder and Joyce Grenfell, did shows in the hospital.

But the most radical measure he took was that he insisted that, as soon as the patients could, they should 'be acclimatised to the people of East Grinstead'.

He sent the patients to the bars and cafes of the town, but first he called meetings of local residents, to explain to them the importance of welcoming the burned and wounded, and he went into each place to explain that the injured airmen were coming and how it was vital they were accepted normally, and for locals not to gawp at their injuries. Some of the airmen couldn't walk, so they were wheeled on beds to the outside of pubs, where other customers would pass beer out of the window to them.

He invited residents into the hospital so they would get to know the patients, so they'd stay positive about what life would be like once they left, confident they wouldn't be stared at because of their injuries. And because of all this, East Grinstead became known as The Town That Does Not Stare.

The success rate of the ward was extraordinary. There wasn't a single case of suicide among the thousands of patients and almost all that survived their severe injuries were able to integrate into society.

What the Guinea Pig Club seemed to embody wasn't just that there is a link between mental and physical health, but that the two combine to determine a person's condition so fully, that it isn't possible to treat one without treating the other.

*

The spirit of Archibald McIndoe persists in every area of medicine – in theory. At the early meetings with consultants, I was asked about my living situation; if I was on my own, how my house was set up and which family members were around me.

I thought this was incidental chat before the serious discussions about masks and radiotherapy. But when I met the medical team after the treatment had ended, they told me these conversations are part of their assessment as to how you will cope and whether you will complete the treatment.

If it's possible you'll be overcome by despair and a sense of hopelessness, by a terror of masks or a fear of eviction when you can't afford the rent, they need to know that in advance. It would be as absurd to ignore the mental state of the patient as it would be to take no notice of the size of their tumour.

So the woman who calls offering to help fill in forms, the extra receptionist that makes it more likely you'll be smiled at when you arrive, the machine that can play a choice of music during the blasts of radiation and the team that curates the art are part of the medical process: as critical in healing patients as the chemo and the drips, as vital as Archibald McIndoe's beer and pretty nurses.

*

Two days before my operation, the troops of Hamas broke into a music festival and murdered over 1,000 Israelis, taking around another 250 as hostages. On top of the horror for those directly involved, the inevitable destruction that would follow and the terrifying global consequences, I thought, *This is really unhelpful timing for me.*

I had shut out as much unpleasantness as possible from the outside world while I had this disease to concentrate on, and now a massive historic event exploded a few hours before I was to be wheeled into an operating theatre. They'd done it on purpose, the bastards.

Over the next few months I consciously and selfishly put aside all the thoughts that tried to creep in about this atrocity and the slaughter in Gaza that followed. Until one afternoon, when one of the most sympathetic of all the nurses on the radiotherapy team was examining me, and I saw she was wearing a small enamel Palestine flag badge.

'I like the badge,' I said.

She told me this badge had inspired 'so many fascinating discussions', in which 'I've learned so much from so many people'. For around 20 minutes she described some of these conversations, with people who did or didn't support the Israeli action, or who had no idea of what lay behind any of it.

The hospital had received no complaints about the badge, she said, and the management were happy that she wore it.

It was by far my favourite 20 minutes of the day (though it wasn't a high bar).

Another major story of the winter was the crisis in the NHS, which was, as it often appears to be, 'on its knees'.

There was the severest shortage of staff, which wasn't helped by the declining living standards of nurses, which seemed even more poignant as it was so soon after the nation had applauded them every week during the Covid lockdown.

It would be hard to ignore this news story. There would be an irony in saying, 'I don't have time to bother with the news about traumas within the NHS because I'm too busy being dependent on treatment from the NHS.'

Because the problem with cutting off the outside world is that eventually you're forced to accept you *are* the outside world.

Throughout the winter there were days of strikes by sections of the staff. Sometimes appointments would be rearranged or delays explained as 'obviously it's difficult at the moment, with the strikes'.

My original operation was postponed because of the strike, and many of the patients I met must have had so many plans sent astray by them.

I was assured my course of radiotherapy wouldn't be affected and felt slightly guilty that the trade union action, which I supported, might be compromised by radiologists continuing to blast me with radiation on strike days.

I'm sure that somewhere on social media there's someone who will angrily tell me I should have carried out my trade union duty and stopped having treatment, because if the comrades of the Spanish Civil War were prepared to die for the cause of the working class, I should have done too.

Just as you never realise, when you're at school, that teachers are human beings with stresses and normal lives and it feels slightly surreal if you see them on a Saturday in a shop with their family, the same is true of doctors and nurses. It felt slightly odd when Philomena told me as she removed a cannula that she was looking forward to getting home, though she needed two buses and the second one had been playing up lately.

One of them might take your blood pressure, giggle with you about a man who tried to walk down Tottenham Court Road still attached to his drip, then tell you they're leaving nursing because they can't afford to stay, not since the landlord put the rent up again.

Maybe the landlords are sorting out an efficient system. If they all put their rents up so much that the cancer patients can't afford to go in for treatment and the nurses can't afford to stay treating anyone, it will all work out perfectly.

*

A series of reports was commissioned into practices in the health service, following disasters in which patients were found to have been treated with neglect. One of them, 'Reforming the Culture of Healthcare: The Case for

Intelligent Kindness', concluded, 'The more attentively kind staff are, the more their attunement to the patient increases; the more that increases, the more trust is generated, there is a reduction in anxiety and the better the outcomes.'

So if the nurse that takes your temperature and the porter that wheels you round the ward engage with you and see you as a person rather than a unit, not only does that liven up your day, it makes it more likely you'll get better, as Archibald McIndoe understood.

On the other hand, a staff that's perpetually stressed about providing the most basic items because their pay has declined will find it harder to act in an attentively kind way, I would imagine.

The outside world that I was trying to cut myself off from had been dominated for many years by the view that for any service or business to operate in the most efficient way, the people in charge had to be motivated, at least in part, by the desire for profit.

This was the antithesis of the philosophy that led to the creation of the NHS, that it should be motivated by a collective responsibility to make the population as healthy as possible, and that leaving health to the demands of profit was inefficient and immoral.

So from the 1980s onwards, the NHS has been an anomaly in British society. It's largely accepted that every other area of life should be run by the demands of business, but most people are adamant that the health service must remain outside this rule. These ideologies are bound to come into conflict. 'Reforming the Culture of Healthcare' commented on this, saying, 'The active promotion of a competitive market economy ... works against the idea of an integrated service that prioritises the need of vulnerable patients, and can insidiously affect the attitudes, feelings and relationships of staff.'

Throughout my time dependent upon the health system, I can't think of any moment in which the motivation for my care was driven by profit. The people who operated on me, investigated me, beamed as they told me, 'This is the 'Rolls-Royce of scans,' felt defeated as they couldn't insert a cannula or proud that they'd discovered a back-door vein, who explained the lymphatic system or the evolutionary role of vocal cords, were propelled by an enthusiasm for knowledge and for life.* I'm sure they all wanted to earn enough money to enjoy their own life, but none of them – up to the highest level – were driven by the compulsion to sell products, increase share prices or float their lecture on the lymphatic system on the stock exchange.

But the NHS has to buy its medicines and equipment and buildings from companies that do have to make a profit. They employ staff from agencies and have coffee shops in their reception areas and get biopsies delivered by companies that answer to shareholders.

And they're funded and ruled by governments whose priorities are not always to fund this island of unprofitability.

As I was awaiting my scan results, a biography of ex-prime minister Liz Truss called *Truss at 10* was published,

* During a meeting with a speech therapist about my battered epiglottis, I was told with enthusiastic delight that the main function of the vocal cords was to protect the airways. To do this most efficiently they vibrate, and it was a happy side-effect of this vibrating that enables us to speak.

written by Sir Anthony Seldon, who had access to many of those who were closest to her during her short reign. Along with her chancellor Kwasi Kwarteng, she had announced a budget containing £45 billion of tax cuts, mostly for the wealthy, which was considered so daft that her government imploded.

Sir Anthony wrote that one of her senior advisers, Alex Boyd, 'was told that Truss and Kwarteng were thinking they could still sort out the black hole with severe cuts', including 'stopping cancer treatment on the NHS'.

Still, we all have to make sacrifices and it's only fair, if £45 billion had been handed out in tax cuts, that it's paid back by the most privileged in society, which is people who've got cancer.

If this unusual way of funding tax cuts had been brought in as she supposedly suggested, it would have been enacted just in time for my diagnosis the following summer. I hope I'd have seen the funny side.

Maybe then chemo could be sold at Costa Coffee by the cup. Perhaps the insertion of a PEG into the stomach could be franchised to Pimlico Plumbers, who will bash it into your stomach with a hammer for £65 an hour or part of an hour plus parts. This was the outside world I was trying to block out as I came up for breath between the deep inhalations of steam that flickered across the co-codamol, the laxative and box upon box of Fortisip nutrition bottles, made by Nutricia, whose agents kept delivering them, eager to plonk another pile on my doorstep when I didn't have enough of a voice to stop them.

After the meeting with the dietician, when I was assured

I could return to normal eating, I asked what I should do with the hundreds of bottles arranged around my kitchen. 'You'll have to chuck them out,' she said. 'They don't tend to take them at food banks, and you can't return them. The company gets paid by the NHS for every box they deliver, whether they're used or not. That's the trouble.'

Twenty-One

That's Life

It's quite common for people who have had a disease such as cancer to say they've had such a wealth of experiences through their treatment, considered so many ideas and developed such deep friendships with so many people and strengthened their ties to those they love, that they're actually glad it happened. So, am I glad that cancer happened to me? Of course I'm fucking not.

Similarly, while I'm sure the spirit of the Blitz must have been profoundly heartwarming, providing the most poignant moment of so many lives, I still feel the rise of Hitler and the Second World War were, on the whole, episodes the human race could have done without.

But it is true that in adversity you reach places that bring the most extreme emotions in all directions. Things I knew in theory I now know for real.

I knew in theory that you should appreciate every day, but now I *feel* it. There's a tingle of delight that I used to sense only at life's most celebratory moments – like when the band you've gone to see plays the introduction to your favourite song, or the instant you're in bed with your partner and realise *Ah, we're* both *up for it tonight*. But now I get these feelings most days – at the realisation there's snooker on the television, at the acrobatics of a random squirrel or the smile of the woman in Sainsbury's who arrives to unlock the broken-down self-service checkout machine.

Conversely, the day after Donald Trump was re-elected as president, I prepared to recline into a depressed stupor, but it never came. Instead I inhabited an anaesthetised helplessness, with no twisting, rasping suction of the internal organs that I used to drown in after a deep disappointment that was beyond my control. It wasn't that I cared less than before, but as there was nothing I could immediately do about it, to get over-stressed seemed counter-productive. I felt almost stoic. I'm sure Marcus Aurelius would have felt the same if Donald Trump had become emperor of Rome.

Maybe these sensations are a result of being forced to consider the finality of life. Because that finality is non-negotiable. There's no court of appeal. You can't ask a union rep or your local MP to write that it really isn't fair that you will die so you hope that fate will recognise this and urgently reconsider.

Because the decisions you make and the emotions you feel are altered by this acceptance, just as a football team that's 1–0 down with three minutes to go doesn't waste time pretending to be injured and not bothering to go forward, because they're aware that time is limited.

To put this another way, if you find yourself with a potentially lethal illness, or you suspect you may one day die, it may be worth thinking about the Russian novelist Dostoyevsky.

Because in 1849 he was arrested for being part of a group that the Tsarist government decreed was subversive and sentenced to death by firing squad. He prepared for his execution until he was reprieved five minutes before he was to be shot.

He described the point at which his life expectancy got down to five minutes, saying he allotted one minute each to think about five separate subjects, memories or people.

I wonder how much of his five minutes he allotted to thinking about the bloke who cut him off as he was turning left onto the A23. Or to how he's never forgiven his brother-in-law for doing a shoddy job when he laid a concrete driveway, or to the anonymous person who called him a 'thick muppet' on Facebook.

We all know, in theory, that spending our time and emotions and sensitivities on issues like these is criminally pointless, but after a glimpse at mortality we feel it.

There is another set of ideas that seems obvious from a year as a cancer patient, which may be true of any trauma. You can 'think' your way to a more peaceful, loving life by dealing with your own emotions and responses, but only within the limits imposed by the world around us.

It's much easier for me to stay calm about Donald Trump than it would be if my family was being deported by him.

I can take comfort in the immense kindness and generosity of the National Health Service because there *is* a National Health Service.

Accepting you can't change what is beyond your control is only a positive outlook if you also commit yourself to try to change what you can try to change.

The NHS was created by people who were dedicated to converting their love and selflessness into an actual physical institution. There are many individuals, corporations and political forces who are dedicated to undermining it, so that love and selflessness would no longer be available to everybody as it is now.

They need to be fought.

*

There was a point during my meeting with Dr Oikonomou, in which he outlined his plan for my treatment, when he said, 'I know you're a comic so we must preserve your voice. But these treatments are not as harsh as they were in the old days.'

He was obviously talking about a time long ago, when they probably dealt with cancer in the neck by pulling the tumour out with a corkscrew.

At the end of the meeting, he mentioned again that the treatment was more precise and less abrasive than the 'old days', adding, 'because that was five years ago'.

Five years ago was the old days! When England lost to Croatia in the World Cup semi-final, when Theresa May was prime minister, when Drake was the best-selling musician in the world, as long ago as THAT.

This is the pace at which the treatment for disease is advancing. It's the pace at which science is allowed to advance. Because science depends on resources being made available for research. And it depends on a willingness for science to be valued at all.

For example, the five years that Dr Oikonomou referred to included the biggest global health scare for a century, during which an equally global movement of 'anti-vaxxers', dedicated to ignoring scientific evidence, was born, and the president of the United States suggested disease could be overcome by drinking bleach.

This was when you could hear someone insist they weren't going to have the Covid vaccine because 'You don't know what's in it', while you're thinking, *But I've seen you buy a kebab from a van at the side of the road at one in the morning.*

Or we were told Bill Gates of Microsoft was placing chips into the vaccine to control our minds. I wanted to reply that I had some sympathy with this, as my mum, in her nineties, was one of the first to be offered the jab. And she was fine for a few hours, but in the evening she went up her road knocking on every door, trying to sell Microsoft Word family packages for £69.99 a year.

But, as with many apparently irrational theories, there's a nugget of sense at their centre. The pharmaceutical companies are massive corporations whose prime motive is profit, so they will spend more on advertising than on research.

Addressing these issues is complex, requires patience and an understanding that not everyone who disagrees is an idiot or a fascist.

It's possible that once your life has been saved by an army of physicians, friends, carers and radiologists, you're better equipped to conduct these debates and battles that propel society in sometimes baffling directions.

Because I can hardly argue now that that kindness and generosity are only practised by people who I agree with about social and political ideas. I received unsolicited help from so many quarters, from nurses with a Palestinian badge to generals in the British Army, from porters I'd marched with against global capitalism to 1970s comics who went to Margaret Thatcher's election rallies, from personal friends of Tony Blair, from Christians and atheists, from bald East Londoners who read the *Daily Mail*, from those I was once in love with and those I was still in love with, from family members who couldn't really understand because they were nearly two or nearly one hundred but they tried their best.*

Like almost all of us, these people are a complex, exhilarating cocktail of emotions and beliefs, but with all of them, underlying is a visceral sense of humanity, with an innate compassion that is beyond dispute. The blossom of the bushes I see may not be as blossomy as the one Dennis Potter saw, but it's definitely more blossomy than it was before.

I am immensely grateful for the abundance of innate compassion sent my way during my cancer episode, not only because it saved my life but because it creates a world that makes our lives worth saving.

*

Physically, I carry a few scars from my treatment. My swallowing mechanism is damaged, possibly forever, so it takes 40 minutes to eat a simple meal and I still can't taste much. My vocal cords are battered so that it's hard to reach more than a handful of notes. My hearing has declined so that I often drift out of conversations as I struggle to make sense of anything being said. (Matthew assures me this is due to inflammation of the Eustachian tube.)

There are exercises and processes I can go through to

* In November 2024 I went to Worcester with all the family, to my mum's 100th birthday party, an afternoon tea at a hotel where the waiters wore bow ties. I expected her to overflow with emotion about my recovery by saying, 'It's a good job you lived, dear, otherwise some of these sandwiches would go to waste.'

minimise these problems, which I take part in. But I don't feel bothered or frustrated by any of it, as it all seems so minor compared to the vast symphony of ideas and emotions that have been thrown up by the bomb that exploded that morning as I was shaving.

The leopard has been taken away. I don't miss it, but I have a strange affection for the adventures it brought me. Sometimes I see something that was chewed up by the leopard and I'm glad it's gone and a bit grateful.

The world can appear to be spiralling ever more uncontrollably to catastrophe, but despite this, to me it seems a little bit warmer, a little bit kinder and a little bit more hopeful than it ever did. And while I never want to see the bloody thing again, I'd like to thank the leopard for that.

Acknowledgements

First of all I would like to thank the people who made this book possible by keeping me alive.

One of the most important qualities any writer must develop is the ability to stay alive long enough to write the book they're writing. This is a point that's often ignored by the academics and people who run writing courses that promise to teach you how to compose a majestic work. Even Stephen King, in his classic book on writing, forgets to mention it.

I wish I knew all their names but I can start with Dr Kokinakis, who studied my ultrasound scan, Dr Oikonomou, who told me I'd live, the consultants Dr Mendes and Dr Vaz, Mustafa, the man who looked like Mustafa, the talented doctor and communicator Mike Elliot, Kate in chemo with her secret vein, Rachel and Steph at speech therapy, Ruheena, Cat the doctor, Cat the dentist, Zainab, the Slovak lymphoedema doctor, the radiotherapists, Jon the doctor, the rest of the speech therapy team, the radiotherapists, receptionists at radiotherapy, the dietician who explained the evolutionary function of the vocal cords, the ear test people, the lovely woman from Nutricia who showed me how to use the syringe, the many nurses who took my blood, the chemotherapy team, the surgeons who fitted my PEG, the people who made my mask, Terry the socialist porter, the nurse who told me I was having the 'Rolls-Royce of scans', the nurses who received my cardboard pot of wee, the anaesthetist I told I was 'famous', the hundreds of nurses I encountered, even the agency nurse who gave me a morphine tablet having forgotten he'd already given me one ten minutes earlier.

I would like to thank all the nurses and doctors who poked a camera up my nostril and round the corner, then down into my throat, a route that, like Mount Everest, was unexplored until one brave soul ventured there, but then became trampled on again and again until it was barely worth a mention.

I would like to thank the multitude of people who rolled me over and took my blood pressure or whacked a machine so it showed a different number, who mopped up the sick of the bloke in the next bed before it stank too much, who wheeled the Polish man outside for his cigarette.

Then there are so many people who kept me going spiritually: Angela Barnes and Matt, Seann Walsh, John and Mark from the cricket team, Dave and Jim the long-suffering fellow Palace fans, Dave and Georgia the wonderful jazz musicians, Pete Graham, Rhod Gilbert and Sian, French Fatima (*LA biopsie*), James Gill, Monica Nash, Andy Zaltzman, Dan Norcross, Richard and Carl and the fine people at BBC Radio (who must have been thinking 'if he carks it that will be a right headache for our schedules'), Phill Jupitus, Mel Hudson, Nick Revell, Rosie Holt, Nick Hancock, Daniel Kitson, Elis and Issy, Mike and Michelle, Sarah from Cornwall, Lisa and Baz and the Khorsandi family and all the people of whom I will think *Oh SHIT, I forgot to thank them*, resulting in a rift that goes on for several generations.

Thanks to Michael Rosen for sending me his magnificent book *Getting Better*, which saw me through some tricky days in hospital, along with the very entertaining autobiography of Bob Monkhouse, one more example of the classic Rosen/Monkhouse combination.

In particular, thanks to the saintly Paul and Vissy and Pete and Kate and Hugh and Jan, Matthew, Pat, Jules and Jo. And thanks to absurdly optimistic ideal cancer companion Matt Forde.

And, in special particular, thanks to Elliot and Eloise and Rae and Shappi.

Thanks so much to Robyn, who had the idea of the book as soon as she read I wasn't well. Just as a comic can't help but think *What's the joke in this?* in every situation, a publisher must think *Is there a book in this?* I'm very glad she did. But thanks also for her advice on which bits to include and which pointless bits to leave out.

Thanks to Emily Martin and David Bamford and Jess Anderson. Thanks to James Jones for the cover design.

And thanks to Aristotle and Leonardo da Vinci and Madame Curie and all the people over thousands of years who have worked out how the body works, and all the millions of people who have battled for a world in which the profits of a few are considered less important than the health and jollity of human beings.